thefacts

Schizophrenia

D0870158

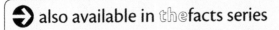 also available in thefacts series

the**facts**

Schizophrenia

FOURTH EDITION

STEPHEN J. GLATT
Director, Psychiatric Genetic Epidemiology & Neurobiology Laboratory
(PsychGENe Lab)
Associate Professor of Psychiatry and Behavioral Sciences, Neuroscience
and Physiology, and Public Health and Preventive Medicine
Associate Director, Psychiatry Research
SUNY Upstate Medical University
Syracuse, New York
USA

STEPHEN V. FARAONE
Distinguished Professor of Psychiatry and of Neuroscience and Physiology
Director, Child and Adolescent Psychiatry Research
SUNY Upstate Medical University
Syracuse, New York
USA

MING T. TSUANG
University Professor, University of California;
Lewis Judd Endowed Chair in Behavioral Genomics;
Distinguished Professor of Psychiatry and Director,
Center for Behavioral Genomics, Department of Psychiatry,
University of California, San Diego
USA

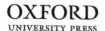

OXFORD
UNIVERSITY PRESS

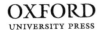

OXFORD
UNIVERSITY PRESS

Great Clarendon Street, Oxford, OX2 6DP,
United Kingdom

Oxford University Press is a department of the University of Oxford.
It furthers the University's objective of excellence in research, scholarship,
and education by publishing worldwide. Oxford is a registered trade mark of
Oxford University Press in the UK and in certain other countries

First Edition Published in 1982
Second Edition Published in 1997
Third Edition Published in 2011
Fourth Edition Published in 2019

Impression: 1

Published in the United States of America by Oxford University Press
198 Madison Avenue, New York, NY 10016, United States of America

British Library Cataloguing in Publication Data

Data available

Library of Congress Control Number: 2018956187

ISBN 978–0–19–881377–4

Printed and bound in Great Britain by
Clays Ltd, Elcograf S.p.A.

Foreword

A diagnosis of schizophrenia can be overwhelming both for the individual and for family members. One of the main problems with schizophrenia is the widespread misunderstanding and falsehoods about what it is and what it means. Around the time of receiving the diagnosis, families often need information but can find the information given by mental health professionals during treatment visits too much to remember. What is needed is a resource that can be accessed whenever family members need it.

All too often today the first port of call is the internet, but as the internet is not moderated or edited in any way the information can be of high quality and can also be misleading. This is why the book by Glatt, Faraone, and Tsuang is so important. There are a few books out there for families, but this book appears unique in that it steps through the important issues of what schizophrenia is—and what it is not—in simple language, thus dispelling myths and misperceptions.

All the time the book is solidly embedded in the research literature and explains what the body of studies over the years have now informed us about this disorder. The various chapters cover the symptoms that can emerge and how the diagnosis is made, with descriptions of the various subtypes of schizophrenia. The authors explain the numerous studies that have informed us about how common schizophrenia is across the world, the genetic basis of the disorder, and the effect of the environment, followed by treatment options and outcome. The final chapter addresses the important role that those living with schizophrenia and their families can do to improve the outcome.

This book will be a hugely important resource of knowledge and information for families affected by schizophrenia.

Ian Paul Everall
Executive Dean
Institute of Psychiatry, Psychology, and Neuroscience
King's College London

Preface

The primary purpose of this book is to provide the lay reader with an introduction to the current state of scientific knowledge regarding the brain disorder known as schizophrenia. As evidenced by the reduced interval at which we are issuing this latest edition (7 years, as opposed to 14–15 for prior editions), things are changing rapidly in the field and facts are accumulating at an unprecedented rate. Without in any way seeking to exclude the professional reader trained in psychiatry or any other branch of medicine or other mental health professionals, we are primarily concerned with helping persons affected with schizophrenia, their relatives, close friends, caregivers, and other acquaintances understand the condition more fully.

To accomplish this aim, we must necessarily employ some specialist terms from the vocabulary of mental health. In doing so, however, we have attempted to adhere to two guiding principles: technical terms will always be clearly defined, and we shall endeavour to steer clear of the use of jargon and 'buzz words' within the discipline of mental health—that is the kind of semi-slang words that professionals in any field use among themselves as a convenient shorthand for more cumbersome terms with meanings that are mutually understood. One example of this, which has changed since the first editions of this book, is our attempt to describe the facts as they pertain to 'individuals with schizophrenia', rather than 'schizophrenics', as we understand these individuals now as suffering from and living with a brain disorder rather than being defined by it. In this latest version, we have also restricted the use of the term 'schizophrenia patients' to instances where we are clearly describing past cases who were patients, or in contexts where diagnosing and treatment are discussed, since not all individuals with schizophrenia are patients or medically diagnosed and treated at all points in their illness.

Concerning references to research in the book, we have kept these to a minimum, partly for reasons of space, but more so to promote easy reading and facilitate readers' processing of 'the facts' as we see them. This is not an academic text and we do not feel it would assist the reader materially to know the source, date, and author of every study used in the book. Naturally, research projects of major importance to the study of schizophrenia—and the investigators who lead them—are identified and documented more fully. Conversely, you may notice that some of the latest and most novel results reported in the scientific literature may not be described fully in the book. Although in many cases we are aware of these studies and are following such developments closely, we have restricted our discussion to topics about which enough is known and enough has been reliably reproduced that they deserve mention in a book subtitled 'the facts'.

Stephen J. Glatt and Stephen V. Faraone, Syracuse, New York
Ming T. Tsuang, La Jolla, California
2018

Endorsements

"*Schizophrenia: The Facts* provides much needed insight into one of the most misunderstood psychiatric disorders. The authors do a remarkable job of explaining the myriad of neurobiological elements surrounding this complicated disease in a manner that is easy to read and tangible for all audiences. This book will surely be a beneficial tool for individuals and families impacted by schizophrenia who constantly struggle to find the answers and solutions to the many challenges the disease poses."

Evelyne Tropper
President, NAMI-NYS

"An essential read for anyone interested in or concerned about schizophrenia and mental disorders in general. The book seamlessly incorporates basic knowledge with new insights derived from cutting-edge research in plain language that is enjoyable for both newcomers and professionals in the field."

Wei J. Chen
Distinguished Professor,
Institute of Epidemiology and Preventive Medicine,
Former Dean, College of Public Health,
National Taiwan University

"I am convinced that this book has an important role to play in helping society and individuals overcome schizophrenia, written to be easily understood by everyone."

Hiroshi Yoneda
Professor of Psychiatry,
Osaka Medical College

"An indispensable source: this book is approachable and readable for professionals, patients, and the public."

Xiaogang Chen
Professor of Psychiatry,
Central South University

Acknowledgements

Preparation of this book was supported in part by grants R01MH085521, R01MH101519, and R01AG054002 from the U.S. National Institutes of Health, and a Katowitz/Radin Young Investigator Award, an Independent Investigator Award, and the Sidney R. Baer, Jr. Prize for Schizophrenia Research from NARSAD: the Brain and Behavior Research Foundation, awarded to Dr Glatt. Dr Faraone was supported by grant R01MH101519 from the U.S. National Institutes of Health. Dr Tsuang was supported by the Lieber Prize for Schizophrenia Research from NARSAD: the Brain and Behavior Research Fund, and grant R01MH085560 from the U.S. National Institutes of Health.

Acknowledgements

Contents

1

What is schizophrenia?

> ## ➔ Key points
>
> ◆ Schizophrenia is a serious mental illness involving changes in thought patterns, emotions, behaviours, and ways of observing the outside world.
>
> ◆ Schizophrenia is probably not one disorder, but a range or 'spectrum' of related disorders that vary in symptoms, severity, and outcome.

Many who pick up this book will be learning about schizophrenia for the first time, either because someone they care about has recently been diagnosed, or purely out of academic interest. As such, we aim to paint a very clear and basic picture of the disorder, and avoid jargon as much as possible (though sometimes this cannot be avoided). The first impression many people get about schizophrenia, however, is formed before they ever meet someone with the disorder, through exposure in films, television, or literature. Some of these portrayals are fair and accurate depictions of particular aspects of schizophrenia, and may be useful to review in combination with this book to help the reader develop a fuller picture of the disorder (though none is perfect in all regards). For example, some aspects of John Nash's struggles with schizophrenia in the film *A Beautiful Mind*, and those of Nathaniel Ayers in *The Soloist*, ring true with these individuals' first-person accounts of the disorder. The reality of schizophrenia has also been reasonably well captured in fictional films such as *Clean, Shaven; Donnie Darko*; and *The Fisher King*. Yet, far more commonly schizophrenia is portrayed in an unrealistic and unflattering light by authors and screenwriters, which adds to the stigma and negative views of the disorder held by many who have no first-hand experience of the illness. We will cover some examples of these faulty depictions later in the chapter 'What is not schizophrenia', but here, let us continue to describe the main facts about the disorder.

Please keep in mind that schizophrenia is one of the most complicated and variable human disorders. Although this is a textbook on schizophrenia, there are no 'textbook cases' of schizophrenia. As such, you may sometimes find yourself reading these facts and thinking, 'that doesn't sound like what I've seen or experienced'. We try to paint as broad a picture of schizophrenia as possible to provide the reader with the best chance of recognizing and understanding schizophrenia when they see it. We use anecdotes about cases to illustrate features of the disorder, but these may not be relevant to the schizophrenia that you have seen. The form of schizophrenia that you see or experience may only exhibit some of these features. Thus, these are the facts on schizophrenia as a whole, but not all facts pertain to all individuals with the disorder.

Schizophrenia is a mental illness with major impacts on affected individuals, their families, and society. Affected individuals show a wide range of problems with their ability to see, hear, and otherwise process information from the world around them (i.e., **perception**). They may also have disruptions in their normal thought patterns, emotions, and behaviours. For many people with schizophrenia, problems with such basic aspects of life can be crippling. They can lead to lifelong disability, repeated stays in the hospital, and difficulty maintaining family and social bonds. Social relationships are often disrupted by the individual's withdrawal and inability to communicate, along with bouts of disruptive behaviour. Families are burdened by the strain of caring for a mentally ill relative and the stigma of mental illness. Because the disorder is so severe and common, schizophrenia is now seen as a major public health concern.

Schizophrenia is a very complex disorder in both its **aetiology** (causes) and its **clinical presentation** (symptoms). Although the illness has been studied for over 140 years, we have much to learn about its causes, course, and treatment. However, the rate of progress has sped up in the last 40 years. Some of these advances come from better methods used to study the disorder, such as brain imaging and molecular genetic tools. Another source of our better understanding is the continued improvement of the diagnostic criteria for schizophrenia. Our current view sees schizophrenia as a point—or endpoint—on a *range* or *spectrum* of abnormal psychology instead of a distinct disease. This view has changed the way in which other questions about the disorder are framed.

The notion of a '**spectrum**' of schizophrenias, including schizophrenia and a number of related—but generally milder—conditions, is not new. The concept was advanced by Dr Eugen Bleuler, who foreshadowed our current view in his 1911 work *Dementia Praecox* or *The Group of Schizophrenias*. We now know that schizoaffective disorder, and schizotypal, paranoid, and schizoid personality disorders, share some symptoms and causes with schizophrenia. This knowledge has helped the search for shared risk factors and treatments. In turn, our ever-increasing knowledge of the basis of schizophrenia has helped understand these other schizophrenia spectrum disorders.

2

What are the symptoms of schizophrenia?

> ### ➲ Key points
>
> ◆ Hallucinations of hearing voices, delusions of being controlled by others, blunting of emotions, and lack of insight are some common schizophrenia symptoms that cut across all cultures or languages.
>
> ◆ Positive symptoms of schizophrenia refer to those features that are *added* to the normal range of behaviour, such as hallucinations and delusions, not to helpful or beneficial qualities of the disorder.
>
> ◆ Negative symptoms refer to the *loss* of normal behaviours. These include affective blunting (inability to show emotion), alogia (lack of speech), avolition (lack of will to interact with the world), anhedonia (loss of ability to feel pleasure), asociality (preference to be alone), and catatonia, which is a group of four cognitive and motor symptoms.
>
> ◆ Negative symptoms are often more difficult to spot and treat than positive symptoms. Compared to positive symptoms, they are less disruptive to others but are just as disabling to affected individuals.

Schizophrenia symptoms fall into two categories: positive and negative symptoms. **Positive symptoms** are behaviours or experiences outside the normal range of human activities. Hearing voices is a good example. **Negative symptoms** are behaviours that are removed from the normal range. A reduced experience of pleasure is a good example. Positive symptoms are prominent during the 'active' phase of the illness, when an affected individual is most disturbed and disruptive. The active phase is the phase that will more often lead to the individual's referral for care. This is often because the affected individual will be doing or saying things that upset or disturb people around them, or at least get their attention and draw concern. For example, an individual with delusions might complain to her spouse that she is being followed by aliens and demand that he help her find a way to stop them. Negative symptoms are most visible during the '**prodromal**' and '**residual**' phases of the illness. The prodromal phase comes before the first active phase (so actually occurs before a diagnosis of schizophrenia is ever made), and a residual phase follows each active phase.

Positive symptoms

This class of symptoms most often includes delusions and auditory, visual, or other sensory hallucinations. Positive symptoms can be divided into **perceptual** (i.e., affecting perception, or the ability to become aware of some stimulus through the senses), **cognitive** (i.e., impacting ways of thinking), **emotional**, or **motor** (physical) signs. Because these symptoms are so easy to recognize, even to the untrained eye, they make up a large part of the layperson's general view of schizophrenia.

Auditory hallucinations are the most common perceptual problems seen in schizophrenia. Many times, these hallucinations take the form of a voice, sometimes making a running commentary on the individual's thoughts or behaviours. Sometimes they take the form of several voices, each talking with the other. Some individuals with schizophrenia have **visual**, **olfactory** (i.e., affecting the sense of smell), or **gustatory** (i.e., affecting taste) **hallucinations**, but these are rare. **Somatic hallucinations** may also occur, in which the altered perception centres at or on the body's organs.

It is important to make a clear distinction between hallucinations, which are perceptions or experiences that occur without a stimulus, and **illusions**, which are perceptions that occur in response to ambiguous stimuli. For example, in response to questions about visual hallucinations, one of our patients said he had seen his dead mother one evening. Further questioning showed that the patient had seen someone who looked like his mother, and the similarity was stronger in the dim light. Although this episode may shed light on the patient's reactions to his mother's death, it was an illusion, not a hallucination indicative of schizophrenia. Visual hallucinations should also not be confused with the 'hypnagogic' imagery that many people experience before falling asleep.

Delusions are false beliefs that are not open to change by reason or experience even though the individual is in an otherwise clear mental state. Delusions are the most common form of thought problems seen in schizophrenia. Interestingly, the *focus* of a delusion usually relates to the affected individual's cultural setting, while the *source* of the delusion is usually personal. In Franz Mesmer's day, individuals with schizophrenia spoke of being controlled by magnetism; 100 years ago, by electricity; and 50 years ago, by television. Now they may speak of being influenced by computers, cellular phones, or the Internet.

Despite the wide variety of delusions seen in individuals with schizophrenia, there are several common themes. For example, individuals who have **paranoid**

delusions report that others are trying to harm them, either emotionally or physically. Like other delusions, these are easy to spot because parts are clearly absurd (e.g., the person may complain that her mother is plotting with the government to prevent her from graduating from high school). In some cases, however, a paranoid belief may appear false because it is unlikely, but may be true. For example, one of our patients had a fear of being attacked by mafia thugs, which was shown to be not delusional but reasonable after careful review of his criminal past.

People with schizophrenia who have **delusions of sin or guilt** believe they are being punished, or should be punished, for something they have done wrong. These delusions may relate to real events or to imagined ones, but even when the event is real, the punishment conjured by the individual far outweighs the severity of the offence (e.g., the individual feels condemned to stay in a closet for the rest of his life because he forgot to mow the lawn for his father). Paranoid and guilty delusions differ in that the paranoid individual believes the persecution they feel is not deserved, whereas the delusionally guilty individual feels the punishment is deserved. Since delusions of sin or guilt are often seen in other mental disorders like mood disorders, individuals with such delusions need to be carefully evaluated for the signs of mood problems seen in depression or bipolar disorder.

Delusions of jealousy involve the belief that a spouse or lover has been unfaithful; such delusions are often hard to judge. If there are no truly bizarre aspects, the delusion can be judged by the affected individual's ability to cite the relevant evidence for and against the delusion. When confronted with evidence against the delusional belief, the truly delusional individual will ignore or explain away such evidence and, as might be expected, even the smallest piece of evidence in support of the delusion is embraced and held dear.

Somatic delusions are often related to somatic hallucinations, in that the source of the delusion is the affected individual's own body. These delusions are usually bizarre and disturbing, and often convey a belief that the individual's body is being harmed or injured. For example, one patient believed his intestines were being eaten by a giant worm. Another was certain he would soon die because his body was rotting from the inside out. These delusions can also occur in other psychiatric conditions, such as depression with psychotic features and delusional disorder, so these disorders must be considered as alternative diagnoses in order to select the right treatment. Somatic delusional disorders are rare and look like other hypochondriacal disturbances in which concerns with and fear about physical health are prominent. The difference lies in the degree of conviction: for the delusional individual, the disease or change in appearance is real, usually bizarre, not grounded in reality, and not open to change.

Individuals with **grandiose delusions** exaggerate their talents and achievements to an unrealistic or even bizarre level. An extreme example would be a patient who claimed to be 'king of the universe' because of his special bond with God. In milder cases, the individual may claim to have unique talents that are not proven (e.g., a patient who claimed to be a great mathematician though his alleged mathematical proofs were meaningless scrawls). Because grandiosity is also a common feature of mania and hypomania, such symptoms should be evaluated to differentiate these conditions from the grandiose delusions of schizophrenia.

If the individual describes false beliefs involving religious or spiritual themes, he may be suffering from a **religious delusion**. The delusional status of a religious belief may be obvious, as in the case of a patient who collected a roomful of grapefruits because she believed they contained the essence of God. However, the delusional status of religious beliefs may be more difficult to establish than that of other types of delusions since a religious belief is not considered delusional if it is consistent with the individual's cultural context. For example, many Jehovah's Witnesses believe in the imminent end of the world. Such a belief would not be delusional if held by a member of that sect, but it might be delusional if expressed by a non-religious individual. In turn, some individuals with schizophrenia may be attracted to unusual religious sects. If this is suspected, then the possibly delusional religious belief should be probed for either a history that came before the individual's association with the sect or parts that are absurd even in the context of the sect.

Other categories of delusions include **bizarre delusions**, in which the content of the belief is illogical and can have no possible basis in fact, and **delusions of being controlled**, in which the affected individual believes that his mind or body is being controlled by an outside source beyond mere persuasion or coercion. Other common delusions involve the belief that an individual's thoughts are being shaped by an outside agency in any number of ways. One example of this type of delusion includes **thought broadcasting**, in which the affected individual believes his ideas are being spoken aloud so that others can hear them. Another example is **thought insertion**, where the individual feels ideas are being inserted into his stream of consciousness by an outside source. The nature of these thoughts is typically unpleasant, and the 'inserted' thoughts may direct the individual to engage in abnormal behaviours. The opposite of thought insertion is **thought withdrawal** and, as its name suggests, this delusion is experienced by the individual as the active removal of thoughts from the stream of consciousness, and the loss of ideas is, again, typically attributed to an outside agency. This process often shows up as **blocking**, which is a sudden stop in the stream of speech.

The catalogue of delusions outlined above shows the amazing diversity of cognitive problems seen in individuals with schizophrenia. The seriousness of a delusion can be rated along five scales: persistence, complexity, bizarreness, behavioural impact, and degree of doubt. The **persistence** of the delusion is measured both as how lasting the belief is and how often the delusion draws upon the affected individual's mental resources. Some individuals with schizophrenia report delusions affecting them daily for months or even years, while others will report delusions that come and go, and which last only several hours at a time.

A delusion's **complexity** refers to the extent to which the delusion forms a complete idea or set of ideas. Sometimes, complexity is quite low, such as when an individual believes that he is the president of the United States but does not develop any elaborate themes or stories associated with his high office. A similar but very complex delusion is illustrated by a patient who believed he was the president of the United States in disguise because of assassination threats by the KGB. He had chosen a job as a bank teller because it would allow him to control the money supply of the country, which was his ultimate source of power. Such a delusion might grow into greater levels of complexity and include friends, relatives, or even strangers who played some role in this unusual story.

Delusions also vary in their levels of **bizarreness** or credibility. Some people with schizophrenia have bizarre delusions that have no credibility whatsoever. Others may express seemingly bizarre delusions that have some level of credibility after considering the person's cultural context. This situation often occurs when the person comes from a deviant cultural context (e.g., the criminal community or an unusual religious sect) and expresses beliefs in line with that context. If a belief is possibly delusional, it is useful to let the affected individual talk about the implications of the belief and associated ideas. With further discussion, a culturally reasonable but unusual belief may blossom into a complex and bizarre delusional system.

A delusion's **behavioural impact** is gauged by its ability to inspire action. At one extreme are individuals who only discuss a delusion when asked, but never perform any related actions. At the other extreme are individuals who constantly preach their delusional beliefs and take extreme, self-damaging actions based on it (e.g., the person who burned his house down because he believed it was haunted by evil spirits trying to kill him). Affected individuals also vary on the **degree of doubt** they have about their delusions. Some believe their delusions with full conviction; others have bizarre ideas that they think *might* be true, but with varying degrees of certainty.

While delusions are the most common thought disruptions seen in schizophrenia, these can be accompanied by **markedly illogical thinking**. For example, an individual with schizophrenia might reason, 'The president of the United States is Protestant; I am Protestant; therefore, I am the president of the United States'. An affected individual's reasoning may also be impaired by a **loosening of associations,** a process by which the individual connects seemingly unrelated concepts to each other. Thought and language usually have a high degree of cohesion that comes from stringing together ideas and/or images that are related to one another in time, space, or by consequences. Loosely related responses to questions are examples of **tangentiality**. In a normal conversation, for example, it is reasonable for an individual to respond to another's description of a fishing vacation by describing his own vacation or asking questions about the other's vacation. An individual with schizophrenia might respond by talking about a tuna fish sandwich that he had the other day. For the individual with schizophrenia, the loose association between a fishing vacation and a tuna fish sandwich justifies the transition. Associations can become so odd and remote that no connection at all is observed between different parts of an affected individual's speech. In the extreme case, persons with schizophrenia speak **word salad**; that is, most of the words in any given sentence appear to have no connection.

In addition to the many cognitive problems seen in their speech and thought processes, persons with schizophrenia also show signs of abnormal emotional regulation. This disruption of emotion takes one of two forms: **inappropriate affect** or **excessive emotional excitement**. Inappropriate affect refers to giggling, self-absorbed smiling, or a mood that is not consistent with expressed ideas. For example, one individual with schizophrenia may grin or chuckle while discussing the death of his brother whom he loved dearly. Another may continually grin or scowl in a bizarre fashion regardless of context. Excessive emotional excitement is often seen in agitated individuals, who *feel* appropriate emotions but, because of delusional thinking or other factors, show these emotions too intensely.

An extreme state of motor excitement seen in some individuals with schizophrenia also qualifies as a positive symptom of the disorder. This agitated state, termed **catatonic excitement**, consists of irregular episodes of uncontrolled and disorganized movement. The individual may gesture excessively and be hyperactive, destructive, or violent. Motor dysfunction also shows as repetitive, apparently meaningless movements known as **stereotypies**. Individuals with schizophrenia also exhibit characteristic mannerisms, consisting of habitual movements that usually involve a single body part (grimaces, tics, moving lips soundlessly, fidgeting with fingers, hand-wringing, or thigh-rubbing).

Negative symptoms

The negative symptoms of schizophrenia are those in which an important or normally occurring part of an individual's behavioural range has become impaired or absent. Just like positive symptoms, negative symptoms affect the cognitive, emotional, and behavioural aspects of life, but do so in the direction of decreased expressiveness and responsiveness. Compared with positive symptoms, negative symptoms are usually more persistent and, in some ways, more devastating; however, negative symptoms do not typically lead to hospitalization because, unlike positive symptoms, they usually do not negatively impact or otherwise impinge upon other people, and therefore do not bring the affected person to the attention of legal or medical authorities. Negative symptoms are more difficult to define and are more difficult to rate reliably, and to treat effectively.

Although most of the thought disruptions in schizophrenia are positive symptoms, some are negative symptoms. The most common are those that reflect a reduced production of thought. **Poverty of speech** means that the individual says very little on his own initiative or in response to questions or situations that would normally evoke speech. The extreme case is **mutism**, in which the affected individual does not speak at all even though he is physically able to do so. **Poverty of content of speech** is seen when the amount of speech is normal but the words convey very little information. **Increased latency of response** refers to a long lag in responses to questions. Blocking occurs when the individual's stream of speech suddenly stops and he cannot continue.

A negative symptom of schizophrenia characterized by a reduction or absence of emotional responsiveness is called **flat, blunt,** or **restricted affect**. Restricted affect is seen in the person's lack of engaging speech, including few vocal inflections or expressive gestures, poor eye contact, decreased spontaneous movements, unchanging facial expression, or a non-responsive mood. Another commonly reported negative mood symptom of schizophrenia is **anhedonia**, or the inability to feel pleasure. Signs of anhedonia are lack of interest in recreation, friendships, sex, or any activity that was previously enjoyable. Diminished emotional responsiveness is also seen in the inability to feel intimacy or closeness with others.

Catatonic stupor is a negative motor symptom of schizophrenia characterized by a decrease of movement and speech. Although rare, some individuals with schizophrenia exhibit **waxy flexibility**, in which they passively allow others to move their limbs into positions that are sometimes uncomfortable, but without ever or rarely moving on their own. **Posturing** (also known as **catalepsy**) refers to holding unusual or uncomfortable positions for long periods during a catatonic stupor. Catatonia in schizophrenia used to be common. Now it is rare.

A related negative symptom of schizophrenia is **negativism**, in which the affected individual strongly resists verbal or physical attempts to engage him in social interaction. Related behavioural impairments are poor grooming and hygiene, inability to persist at tasks, and withdrawal from social activities. The study of social behaviour in people with schizophrenia has shown that the disorder results in a marked loss of the basic behavioural components needed for effective social interaction.

3

How is schizophrenia diagnosed?

⊖ Key points

♦ Many conditions cause symptoms like those of schizophrenia, so it is important that persons with possible schizophrenia get proper medical care. This process helps the clinician figure out how to treat the patient's condition.

♦ Through 'differential diagnosis', the clinician rules out other conditions that could cause the patient's condition, such as encephalitis, drug abuse, epilepsy, or well-defined brain diseases.

♦ Schizophrenia is not a mood disorder. Persons with mood disorders exhibit periods of very high emotional states of euphoria, talkativeness, and high activity (mania), or very low emotional states and feelings of worthlessness (depression).

♦ Delusions occur in both mood disorders and schizophrenia, though they differ greatly between the two. In mania, delusions are often grandiose, while delusions of worthlessness and guilt may be present in depression. In schizophrenia, delusions are usually bizarre or paranoid.

♦ People who have both the symptoms of schizophrenia and the changes of mood found in mood disorders may have a schizoaffective disorder.

The diagnosis of schizophrenia cannot be made based on the results of an objective diagnostic test or laboratory measure, though we and others are working towards this. Instead, clinicians diagnose schizophrenia based on behaviour and psychopathology (including the symptoms described in the previous chapter). These require the subjective interpretation of clinicians, but they can be assessed reliably.

The definitions of major mental illnesses used by clinicians are presented in the Diagnostic and Statistical Manual (**DSM**) of the American Psychiatric Association (in the United States) and the World Health Organization's International Classification of Diseases (**ICD**) in other countries. These definitions are updated from time to time to reflect gains in knowledge, or to reflect modern thinking on the similarities and differences between certain disorders. From one edition to the next, some diagnoses are revised, some are added, and some vanish altogether, only to be replaced or absorbed under other diagnoses.

The diagnostic criteria for schizophrenia as defined by the most recent version of the DSM (DSM-5) include the presence of two or more of the following symptoms: delusions, hallucinations, disorganized speech, disorganized or catatonic behaviour, and negative symptoms. At least one of the two must be delusions, hallucinations, or disorganized speech, while the second symptom type required for diagnosis could be any of the remaining four criteria. The requirement of delusions, hallucinations, or disorganized speech maintains the resemblance of the modern-day diagnosis to that first described by the clinician Emil Kraepelin over a century ago.

Kraepelin's discovery that schizophrenia is marked by a chronic and gradually worsening course is seen in modern-day criteria as well. A DSM-5 diagnosis of schizophrenia requires continuous signs of illness for at least 6 months, during which the individual must show at least 1 month of active symptoms (less if well treated). The diagnosis also requires social or work deterioration over a significant amount of time.

Lastly, the diagnosis requires that the observed symptoms are not due to some other medical condition, including other psychiatric disorders such as bipolar disorder or major depressive disorder. If a full depressive or manic syndrome is seen, the individual would not be diagnosed with schizophrenia unless the mood problems came after the active phase of the schizophrenia syndrome, or were brief in relation to it. Beyond these closely related and easily confused psychiatric disorders, general medical conditions, substance use, and pervasive developmental disorders must be excluded. These exclusions are needed because other conditions mimic the signs and symptoms of schizophrenia.

When these diagnostic criteria are applied well, the reliance on observable changes in behaviour minimizes inferences or 'best guesses', and improves the chance that two separate clinicians can diagnose the same person with the same disorder. In this scheme, there is no room for guessing about potential causes. However, the process of making a diagnosis is not a rote exercise in counting the number of criteria met; sound clinical skill and experience are essential. With structured criteria like those in the DSM, clinical judgement enters into the evaluation of whether the symptoms within a specific, well-defined criterion are present or not. Thus, the use of structured diagnostic criteria in the DSM-V has not reduced the need for clinical judgement; it has merely focused this judgement on the data collection process of the diagnostic work.

Subtypes of schizophrenia

Although Kraepelin originally described schizophrenia as a single disorder, he and his peers also saw that there were many different ways in which schizophrenia appears. Initially, Kraepelin made the distinction between hebephrenic, catatonic, and paranoid subtypes of schizophrenia, and the clinician Eugen Bleuler later added a subtype called simple schizophrenia. The use of the term 'schizophrenic disorders' instead of 'schizophrenia' to describe this illness in the earlier versions of the DSM emphasized this variety of clinical presentations. Five major subtypes of schizophrenia have been recognized in more recent versions of the DSM: paranoid, disorganized, catatonic, undifferentiated, and residual. In the most recent version of the manual (DSM-5), the subtype descriptions have been removed, because research showed that the subtypes were not stable over time, and did not affect treatment decisions or relate to outcomes. Given that these subtypes are no longer used by clinicians, we only describe them briefly here.

The hallmark of **paranoid schizophrenia** is a preoccupation with one or several delusions or persistent auditory hallucinations. The delusions of an individual with paranoid schizophrenia are usually persecutory or grandiose, but other delusions can occur. Many times, the hallucinations experienced by the individual are related to the nature of his delusions. Along with these features, the individual may carry a sense of constant suspicion and may seem tense, guarded, or reserved to the point of vagueness or even mutism. While delusions and hallucinations are almost always seen in individuals with this subtype of schizophrenia, other clinical features, such as hostility, aggression, and even violence, may be present in varying degrees, especially when the disorder is not being treated effectively. Paranoid individuals show only mild, if any, problems with cognition and their chance for a positive long-term outcome is typically better than that of individuals with other schizophrenia subtypes.

As its name suggests, **disorganized schizophrenia** is characterized by muddled or confused speech, disorganized behaviour, and flat or inappropriate affect. The individual with disorganized schizophrenia may voice hypochondriacal complaints and have bizarre thoughts. Often these individuals exhibit bizarre behaviours and suffer from severe social withdrawal. The individual may have fragmentary delusions or hallucinations, but they are never organized and are without a coherent theme. Disorganized schizophrenia shows an early and sudden onset of the illness and usually has a chronic course.

Catatonic schizophrenia was named for the unusual motor problems seen in this group of individuals. Their severe psychomotor disturbances range from negativism, mutism, and rigidity, to a dangerously excitable and agitated state. Movements and mannerisms become stereotyped, and the affected individual may show periods of extreme stupor in which a state of waxy flexibility is observed. Some catatonic individuals rapidly alternate between extremes of stupor and excitement, posing an unpredictable threat to themselves or others. As these abnormal motor states can last for long periods of time, the catatonic individual may become malnourished, exhausted, or develop an extremely high temperature. While catatonic schizophrenia was common many years ago, it is now rare.

Undifferentiated schizophrenia is diagnosed if all criteria are met, but the clinical picture does not fit any of the three subtypes already described.

The **residual schizophrenia** subtype was used to classify those individuals with a history of at least one schizophrenic episode and some residual signs of the disorder, but no active psychotic symptoms. Examples of 'residual signs' of the disorder are features resembling negative symptoms, such as emotional blunting and social withdrawal, or positive symptoms, including illogical thoughts, eccentric behaviour, and a loosening of associations. If delusions and hallucinations are present, they are relatively mild and have little emotion associated with them.

The schizophrenia spectrum

Schizophrenia is a baffling disorder with a wide array of symptoms. The disorder's **heterogeneity**, or lack of consistency from one person to the next, helps schizophrenia avoid any simple explanation, and the similarity of schizophrenia to the psychoses brought on by a variety of medical conditions and abuse of drugs further hurts our efforts to understand this illness. In the 1960s, Seymour Kety was one of the first to propose that schizophrenia, as it was strictly defined, was one condition along a spectrum of mental disorders with varying degrees of severity. By viewing schizophrenia not as an all-or-nothing trait but as one of degrees, Kety provided a framework in which the risk for schizophrenia-like symptoms could vary over a wide range of values, from the totally unaffected person to the severely impaired individual. The spectrum concept illustrates, at the level of clinical presentation, the causal theories of the disorder that also emerged during this time. In a model first proposed by Irving Gottesman and James Shields—the **multifactorial polygenic (MFP) model**—some degree of unseen risk for schizophrenia is present in all individuals. In this model, the degree of risk is set by the small, additive effects of many genetic and environmental risk factors. If the number of factors held by any given person is beyond some threshold level, then that person will develop schizophrenia; if the threshold level is not reached, full schizophrenia is avoided, but some schizophrenia-like symptoms may be seen in a milder form. If no genetic or environmental risk factors are present, the individual shows no signs of any problems along the schizophrenia spectrum (Figure 3.1).

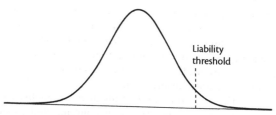

Figure 3.1 Risk Liability Threshold Model. This figure represents the distribution of risk for schizophrenia in the population. In the left or low end of the distribution are those very few among us who have the lowest risk for schizophrenia. Most people, making up the bulk of the middle part of the distribution, have a moderate degree of risk for the disorder, but not enough to put them over a threshold of risk that would cause the disorder. Like the bottom of the distribution, the top or right end of the distribution also contains relatively few people, but these individuals have the most risk factors for schizophrenia, beyond a critical threshold of liability, and will develop the disorder.

The MFP model is consistent with findings that the relatives of individuals with schizophrenia also have a higher rate of schizophrenia-like psychoses, including schizoaffective disorder, schizophreniform disorder, and other psychotic disorders, as well as several personality disorders whose clinical presentations are similar to—but less severe than—schizophrenia. These latter disorders are schizotypal personality disorder, paranoid personality disorder, and schizoid personality disorder. People with these personality disorders do not become psychotic but show unusual behaviours that are similar to but milder than the signs and symptoms of schizophrenia.

Two lines of evidence have defined schizophrenia spectrum disorders. The first is that a disorder should show some clinical similarity to schizophrenia. For example, the suspiciousness of a person with paranoid personality disorder is not delusional, but is similar to a paranoid delusion. The second criterion for inclusion in the schizophrenia spectrum is that a disorder should be more common in families having a member with schizophrenia than in other families. The idea here is that the family member with schizophrenia has a 'full dose' of schizophrenia genes and environmental risk factors, but the member with a spectrum disorder only has a 'mild dose'.

Schizoaffective disorder

According to DSM-V's diagnostic standards, schizoaffective disorder has many symptoms in common with schizophrenia, along with symptoms of unusually high or low mood. In fact, the diagnostic criteria for schizoaffective disorder specify that the same core symptoms of schizophrenia must be satisfied and that delusions or hallucinations must be present, but in addition the mood disturbance must be present for more than half of the total period of illness. Thus, schizoaffective disorder shares more in common with schizophrenia clinically than any other disorder. Of the two subtypes of schizoaffective disorder, the depressive type is thought to lie nearer the schizophrenia spectrum, while the bipolar type is thought to have causes that are closer to that of bipolar disorder; however, there is evidence that both subtypes are on a disease continuum that includes schizophrenia, suggesting that the traditional boundary between schizophrenia and mood disorders may be somewhat artificial and unjustified. This is an important area of active research.

Dozens of family-based genetic studies (including twin and adoption studies) have found a higher-than-average rate of schizoaffective disorder among the biological (but not adoptive) relatives of individuals with schizophrenia, which underscores the importance of a genetic relationship between schizophrenia and schizoaffective disorder. The rate of schizoaffective disorder among family members of people with schizophrenia may be as high as 9%, which is well above the rates of schizoaffective disorder in the general population (less than 1%).

Psychotic disorder, not otherwise specified

In practice, it is not uncommon to come across individuals who are psychotic but do not meet the criteria for schizophrenia or the other differential diagnostic categories mentioned above. Many of these individuals will be diagnosed as having psychotic disorder, not otherwise specified (**NOS**), which is a residual category reserved for such individuals. Examples of psychosis NOS are transient psychotic episodes related to possible environmental or biological events, persistent auditory hallucinations as the only disturbance, and psychoses with confusing or unusual clinical features. Some individuals diagnosed with psychotic disorder, NOS, will eventually be diagnosed with schizophrenia as their disorder evolves.

Schizophreniform disorder

Individuals who meet the criteria for schizophrenia but have only exhibited symptoms for 1–6 months may receive a diagnosis of schizophreniform disorder. Because individuals with schizophreniform disorder meet several diagnostic criteria for schizophrenia, the differential diagnosis of these two related disorders is impractical. Instead, many cases of schizophreniform disorder are coded as 'provisional', meaning that the individual has had symptoms for only 1–6 months but may continue to show symptoms that may eventually qualify the individual for a different diagnosis, such as schizophrenia.

Schizotypal personality disorder

Of several personality disorders that have clinical features in common with schizophrenia, schizotypal personality disorder is the most similar regarding the number of shared criteria and the degree of impairment. This is in part because the diagnosis of schizotypal personality disorder is based on the presence of both social and cognitive problems, which are also central to the diagnosis of schizophrenia itself. In fact, the features of schizotypal personality disorder reflect those of schizophrenia, but with less severity. For example, the ideas of reference, odd beliefs, magical thinking, unusual perceptual experiences, and suspiciousness that characterize schizotypal personality disorder are milder forms of the delusions and hallucinations of paranoid schizophrenia. Likewise, the odd thinking, speech, and behaviour of this personality disorder resemble the similar—but more severe—features of disorganized schizophrenia. Furthermore, the appearance of mood disturbance, the lack of close friends, and the social anxiety commonly seen in schizotypal personality disorder are easily recognizable as diluted forms of the social dysfunction of schizophrenia.

Paranoid personality disorder

Individuals with paranoid personality disorder have a consistent distrust and suspiciousness of others, where evil motives are ascribed to others without sufficient basis. Although paranoid personality disorder shares only this single group of symptoms with schizophrenia, these features are central to the diagnosis of paranoid-type schizophrenia; thus, the inclusion of paranoid personality disorder into the group of schizophrenia spectrum disorders seems warranted.

Schizoid personality disorder

In the same vein, there also appears to be good reason to include schizoid personality disorder in the group of schizophrenia spectrum disorders. The main clinical feature of schizoid personality disorder is a consistent pattern of social dysfunction ranging from lack of social relationships to restricted expression of emotions in interpersonal settings, symptoms that are similar to (but less severe than) the social dysfunction that is a core feature of schizophrenia.

Non-psychotic schizophrenia spectrum conditions have also been studied in this manner to determine their familial clustering with schizophrenia. Several studies have shown that some relatives of individuals with schizophrenia have negative personality traits, such as impaired interpersonal relationships, social anxiety, and a more narrow range of emotional responses. Less frequently, mild forms of thought disorder, suspiciousness, magical thinking, illusions, and perceptual problems have been seen. This set of personality characteristics points to higher rates of schizotypal, schizoid, and paranoid personality disorders among the relatives of individuals with schizophrenia. Among these disorders, schizotypal personality disorder shows the strongest familial link with schizophrenia, with rates of the personality disorder 1.5–5 times higher among the relatives of individuals with schizophrenia than in the relatives of comparison subjects or in the general population. Furthermore, adoption studies show that schizotypal personality disorder has not only a familial relationship with schizophrenia but also a truly genetic link.

Studies of paranoid and schizoid personality disorders have not provided a similar level of evidence for a familial association with schizophrenia. In fact, more than one study has found no increase in the rate of paranoid personality disorder among the first-degree relatives of individuals with schizophrenia when compared to the rates observed in the family members of comparison subjects. Schizoid personality disorder has been found to have a slightly stronger relationship with schizophrenia, but the evidence for a familial link with schizophrenia is still weak overall. Based on the superficial similarities of these two personality disorders to schizophrenia, it is indeed surprising that neither disorder shows a stronger genetic relationship to schizophrenia.

Differential diagnosis of other psychotic disorders

Psychotic disorder due to a general medical condition

A diagnosis of schizophrenia should only be made after careful exclusion of any non-psychiatric medical conditions that can be detected through clinical examination, collection of medical history, or laboratory findings. Schizophrenia-like psychosis is more common in individuals who sustain a closed head injury, for example, and the trauma need not have occurred at any particular brain region; rather, a brain injury of any type may cause such symptoms. Other medical conditions, such as temporal lobe epilepsy, can produce symptoms, such as frank psychosis, that very closely resemble those of schizophrenia.

Substance-induced psychotic disorder

As in the general population, drug abuse has become much more common among individuals with psychiatric disorders over the last four decades. Because so many legal and illegal drugs cause behaviours that are similar to symptoms of schizophrenia, especially psychosis, the differential diagnosis of substance use and schizophrenia based solely on clinical presentation is very difficult. Although the differences between substance-induced psychoses and the psychosis of schizophrenia are subtle, progress has been made in establishing criteria that may distinguish between the two. For example, amphetamine psychosis can be differentiated from paranoid schizophrenia by both the prominence of visual hallucinations and the relative absence of thought disorder with amphetamine use. Compared with schizophrenia, amphetamine psychosis is also more likely to lead to distortion of body image. Other reports, however, suggest that the most common features of amphetamine psychosis are indistinguishable from schizophrenia, so this continues to be an area of active research and debate.

The psychosis produced by the use of lysergic acid (LSD), like that seen with amphetamine, can be differentiated from the psychotic features of schizophrenia based on the increased prevalence of visual hallucinations, and can also be distinguished based on the presence of mystical preoccupation and subtle gaps in logic. LSD-induced and schizophrenic psychoses can further be discriminated by more disorganization of concepts and more excitement, along with less motor retardation and blunt affect, in the drug-induced state. However, just as some have found amphetamine-induced and schizophrenic psychoses to be indistinguishable, some researchers have challenged the generality of any distinctions between LSD-induced psychosis and that of schizophrenia. Attempts have also been made to distinguish between the psychotic symptoms of schizophrenia and the effects of the dissociative compound phencyclidine (PCP), again with mixed results.

A comprehensive review of the available literature suggests that typical substance-induced psychoses are not identical to typical examples of schizophrenia, but that individual features of the two are similar. Thus, despite the best efforts of many researchers, it is quite clear that reliance on symptoms alone is not adequate for differentiating drug-induced conditions that resemble schizophrenia from the disorder itself. When drug histories are unreliable, or when multiple drugs have been abused, clinical features will be even less useful in deriving an accurate diagnosis. Furthermore, if the length of the drug-induced psychotic episode is longer than the duration of drug action, the discriminating power of the criteria outlined above will be quite low. However, if the individual's prior history is relatively normal and the duration of psychosis does not exceed the duration of drug action, then it is reasonable to assume the psychosis is substance induced. We have found that psychotic drug abusers having psychotic symptoms that exceed the duration of drug action but lasting less than 6 months have better pre-psychosis personalities, shorter hospitalization, less need for pharmacotherapy, better prognosis at discharge, and lower familial risks for psychiatric disorders than do psychotic drug abusers whose psychoses exceed 6 months in duration. Thus, it appears that the effective differential diagnosis of schizophrenia and substance-induced psychoses requires adequate observations of the course of the disorder.

Delusional disorder

Although delusional (paranoid) disorder is a rare condition, it is easily confused with paranoid schizophrenia and so must be carefully differentiated from this schizophrenia subtype. Delusional disorder comprises a group of syndromes in which the delusion is the critical shared element; however, individuals with this disorder do not meet all criteria for schizophrenia. The affected individual's delusions are well systematized and logically developed. Before the DSM-5, delusional disorder was called paranoid disorder, but this transition represents the evolution of the diagnostic category to include delusions in which persecution or jealousy is not the main focus. In the differential diagnosis of delusional disorder and paranoid schizophrenia, it is critical to establish the presence or absence of hallucinations. Hallucinations may be a feature of paranoid schizophrenia but are not associated with delusional disorder. Delusional disorder can be further differentiated from paranoid schizophrenia based on the absence of positive symptoms, except the delusion. In further contrast with paranoid schizophrenia, the delusions experienced by the individual with delusional disorder are typically somewhat plausible and not bizarre.

Brief psychotic disorder

The diagnosis of brief psychotic disorder is appropriate for individuals exhibiting classic symptoms of schizophrenia that last for only a short period. To qualify for this diagnosis, symptoms such as disorganized speech, disordered behaviour, delusions, or hallucinations may only be present for a period between 1 day and 1 month. Brief psychotic disorder is usually caused by a profoundly stressful event, in response to which the affected individual becomes overwhelmed with emotional turmoil or confusion. Although the symptoms of this disorder persist for only a limited amount of time, this condition can be severely debilitating and can place the individual at increased risk for harm due to the cognitive impairment, delusional thought structure, and faulty judgement imposed by the disorder. In some cases of brief psychotic disorder, the existence of a personality disorder similar to the schizophrenia prodrome (i.e., vague, less severe schizophrenia-like symptoms) may suggest schizophrenia. Careful examination of the personality structure and observation of the clinical course will clarify this distinction.

Shared psychotic disorder

If an individual presents with a delusion similar in content to one that has been previously established in another individual, a diagnosis of shared psychotic disorder may be made. In many cases of shared psychotic disorder, the two individuals are related to one another and, in their relationship, the first one to become psychotic is often the dominant member of the pair. Shared psychoses usually occur between two individuals, which is why this disorder is also known as *folie à deux*, but they may also occur among members of a large group.

Mood disorders

Differentiating between schizophrenia and major mood disorders with psychotic features can be difficult. Hallucinations and delusions are seen in many individuals with mania or depression, and these features can resemble those of schizophrenia. The two disorders are differentiated in the DSM-V based on the length of the manic or depressive episode. Thus, if the altered mood state is not brief relative to the length of time that core schizophrenia symptoms are present during both the active and residual phases of the illness, a mood disorder may be indicated instead. Of course, knowing the relative duration that a set of symptoms has been present in the course of an illness can be difficult.

To assist the differential diagnosis of schizophrenia and mood disorders beyond the criteria laid out above, a clinician can examine the content of the individual's hallucinations and delusions. If these psychotic features conform to the individual's mood state, a mood disorder is suspected. For example, mania is often marked by grandiose delusions, and depressed individuals often have delusions of sin or guilt. The content of auditory hallucinations may also conform to mood states, and if undertones of joy or despair are seen, these can also help in this differential diagnosis. If the affective tone of hallucinations and delusions is ambiguous or uninformative, and if the affected individual cannot be diagnosed with either schizophrenia or a mood disorder based on other criteria, a diagnosis of schizoaffective disorder is appropriate.

The most efficient way to minimize the improper classification of other disorders as schizophrenia is to collect all the available data on each individual and to recognize that no clinical feature is entirely characteristic of the disorder. If based on a thorough clinical interview, the diagnosis of a psychotic individual is still unclear, it is sometimes useful to collect information about psychiatric illness in biological relatives. Although family psychiatric history is not part of the diagnostic criterion in DSM-V, family, twin, adoption, and molecular genetic studies suggest that a psychotic individual with relatives affected by schizophrenia is more likely to have schizophrenia, whereas one with manic or depressed relatives is more likely to have a mood disorder. Recent work does show, however, that neither set of disorders 'breeds true', and that having either schizophrenia or a mood disorder in the family increases the risk of *both* schizophrenia and mood disorders to other members of the family.

Continued evolution of the diagnosis of schizophrenia and schizophrenia spectrum disorders

A major revision of the DSM (DSM-5) was completed in 2013, and a new version of the DSM may not be anticipated for another decade. Thus, the current diagnostic structure is 'here to stay' for a while. The revision updated the manual based on our evolving understanding of schizophrenia and other disorders. It also brings the DSM criteria more in line with the other major diagnostic and classification system used by much of the world; i.e., the World Health Organization's ICD system, which is presently in its tenth edition.

The changes made to the DSM-5 criteria for schizophrenia were substantial, including most notably the abolition of all five schizophrenia subtypes. This decision was based on clinical practice (the subtypes were not useful) and, more importantly, their heuristic value relative to their validity. In the years to come, clinicians and researchers will set their sights on updating the diagnoses of DSM-5 or redefining the overall structure of the diagnostic system. A major push is being made by the leading public mental health research agency in the United States (the National Institute of Mental Health) to push the concept of spectrums and dimensions of behaviour further from a research effort and more toward a clinical/diagnostic paradigm. Thus, DSM-5 does already include several dimensional scales for rating the severity of symptoms in several domains, including psychosis, anxiety, and others. For psychosis, DSM-5 allows the clinician to rate the severity of deficits in several dimensions: hallucinations, delusions, disorganization, abnormal psychomotor behaviour, restricted emotional expression and avolition, impaired cognition, depression, and mania. Each category of severity is assessed on a four-point scale with reference to the last month. These dimensional ratings are used as added information to go along with the diagnostic judgement of a disorder, but the ultimate diagnosis remains a yes/no decision. With the continued push for research on clinically useful rating scales and dimensions of behaviour, we anticipate that severity rating scales such as that currently used for psychosis may be, in some way, utilized in the identification of schizophrenia as present and at a particular level.

A watershed event for the field would be the inclusion of a psychosis-risk diagnosis in the next version of the DSM. Such a category was considered for DSM-5, but ultimately judged not yet ready for routine clinical use. This diagnosis would be given in situations where an individual exhibits all of the following: (1) delusions, hallucinations, or disorganized speech in reduced form with intact reality testing, but of sufficient severity and/or frequency that it is not discounted or ignored; (2) symptoms must be present in the past month and occur at an average frequency of at least once per week in the past month; (3) symptoms must have begun in or significantly worsened in the past year; (4) symptoms are sufficiently distressing and disabling to the individual and/or parent/guardian to lead them to seek help; (5) symptoms are not better explained by any DSM-V diagnosis, including substance-related disorder; and (6) clinical criteria for any DSM-V psychotic disorder have never been met.

This designation would be a formal recognition that the schizophrenia prodrome is a clinically meaningful and actionable state. Creating a psychosis-risk diagnosis would have important individual and public health benefits, because the identification of the at-risk or prodromal state as a real clinical entity might allow treatment to commence sooner, leading to prevention of illness, reduction of severity and an overall better outcome.

4

What is not schizophrenia?

> ## ⊃ Key points
>
> ◆ Despite common misconception, schizophrenia is not ambivalence (being of two minds or two opinions on a matter), or 'split personality', 'multiple-personality', or dissociative identity disorder.
>
> ◆ Some of the symptoms of schizophrenia can cause it to be mistaken for other disorders such as mood or substance use disorders, so careful differential diagnosis is essential to guide treatment.

The words 'schizophrenia' and 'schizophrenic' are often misused in daily conversation, in literature and film, and even in the popular news media. They mean different things to different people: an attitude of mind, a type of personality, or a psychiatric illness. For example, someone who can't make up his mind, or who has feelings of both love and hate for something, may be falsely called schizophrenic ('ambivalent' is the more proper term). In some cultures, especially in the past, schizophrenia was seen as a sign of possession by an evil spirit or even as a sign of religious superiority. Individuals with schizophrenia were either punished or praised in accord with the beliefs of their culture.

Today, the most common misconception is that a person with schizophrenia has a 'split' personality or multiple personalities. Examples of this in film include *Me, Myself, and Irene*, in which the main character is diagnosed with 'advanced delusionary schizophrenia with involuntary narcissistic rage' instead of what appears to be dissociative identity (formerly known as multiple personality) disorder. Even films that do a decent job depicting schizophrenia can get some aspects wrong; for example, *A Beautiful Mind*, which we earlier cited as a relatively well-done depiction of the disorder, also misses the mark by exaggerating the role of visual hallucinations of full-figure humans in guiding the main character through various and extensive 'missions'.

The correct use of the word 'schizophrenia' is as a diagnostic term used to define a specific mental condition based on clear criteria. As described in our chapters on symptoms and on how schizophrenia is diagnosed, differential diagnosis is essential; that is, determining if the symptoms are really indicative of schizophrenia or of other conditions. Recognizing if mood disturbances (including depression and/or mania), delusions (particularly grandiosity and delusions of sin or guilt), hallucinations, and disorganization are not actually reflective of a mood disorder, substance use disorder, or developmental or neurological disorder is essential, since each type of disorder has a different treatment. Furthermore, it is vital to consider cultural context when determining if behaviour is truly bizarre and qualifies for a diagnosis or is simply normal within the individual's social setting.

When we define schizophrenia appropriately using structured diagnostic criteria, and when we use the word 'schizophrenia' in the right way, it has very specific implications for the treatment of the condition, its course, and our knowledge about its causes. The correct use of this word improves public awareness, diminishes stigma, and leads to better outcomes for people with the disorder. Common and careless use of words such as 'crazy', 'nuts', 'wacko', 'insane', and the like, in conversation or media, do little to encourage those with schizophrenia to seek help. The disorder itself often makes them fearful and isolated; yet we know that people with schizophrenia have the best possible outcome when they seek treatment as soon as symptoms emerge. Improving our language, attitudes, and actions towards people with schizophrenia, especially during the prodromal stage, would create a culture of openness and help-seeking without fear of judgment and stigma, and lessen the impact of the disorder on those with the disorder, their loved ones, and society.

5

How common is schizophrenia?

➔ Key points

◆ International studies show that, with a few exceptions, the prevalence of schizophrenia is similar around the world—between 0.5% and 0.8%.

◆ In reporting the rates of schizophrenia, the term 'incidence rate' is used when estimating the number of new cases in a year. 'Prevalence rate' is used when both old and new cases are counted over a short period.

◆ The lifetime risk for schizophrenia is about 1%, meaning that nearly 1 in 100 people will develop schizophrenia in their lifetime.

How to read and interpret scientific results

To this point, we have been providing consensus descriptions of schizophrenia, what it is and what it is not, and describing the means by which it is detected and diagnosed. In this and later chapters, we present the evidence about the causal factors, treatments, and outcomes of schizophrenia from scientific studies. Such studies sometimes find results that differ from each other due to differences in the methods used or the types of patients that are studied. Random differences in measurement between studies also leads to discrepancies, which is perfectly normal.

How, then, can we come to firm conclusions in the presence of variable results from different studies? Our approach as scientists, and as authors trying to distil the facts, is to always rely on the *preponderance* of evidence, or the best estimate that can be made when putting all the evidence together. Thus, as we present the facts moving forward, we will base our claims on the largest studies available, since these usually give more reliable results than small studies. Whenever possible, we will present the results of analyses that put the results of other studies together using a formal statistical method called '**meta-analysis**'. Thus, instead of comparing and contrasting the results from two or more studies, we will let the reader know the overall result found when all studies were pooled together. In some instances, however, it is instructive to compare and contrast studies because each study tells us something different and uniquely important, and we will point this out when doing so.

Fundamentals of epidemiology

In this chapter, we describe the epidemiology of schizophrenia. **Epidemiology** is a branch of science concerned with the distribution and determinants of illness in the population, and the transmission of illness within families. Two important epidemiologic measures of disease burden in society are **prevalence** and **incidence**. The prevalence of schizophrenia (i.e., the number of affected individuals in the population) has been estimated at least 60 times in 30 different countries (Table 5.1). The prevalence estimates seen in these studies are very consistent, despite cultural differences between samples and the different methods used and timeframes sampled in the studies. These results show that schizophrenia is not specific to one type of culture and that the disorder does not differ much between East and West or between developed and less-developed countries. The lowest estimate of schizophrenia's prevalence was 0.6 cases per 1000 people sampled in Ghana, and the highest prevalence was in Sweden, where 17.0 cases per 1000 were found in one sample. This unusually high prevalence may be due to environmental factors. That sample was a north Swedish isolate separated from the rest of the country where the population is sparse and social stimulation is limited. It has been suggested that such environments may be more conducive to the withdrawn, isolated lifestyle that many individuals with schizophrenia prefer.

As seen in Table 5.2, the lifetime risk for schizophrenia has been estimated at between 0.3% and 2.7%, with an average of just less than 1.0%, a value which, again, has been supported by a recent summary of these and other studies finding a lifetime prevalence of 0.5%. Thus, nearly one of every 100–200 individuals can be expected to develop schizophrenia at some point in their life, according to the best available estimate of the population prevalence.

It is also very useful to know the incidence of schizophrenia, which is the number of new onsets of the disorder that occur in a defined period. Estimates of schizophrenia incidence in ten different countries vary from a low of 0.10 per 1000 to a high of 0.69 per 1000, with an average of 0.35 new cases of schizophrenia per 1000 individuals in a given population per year (Table 5.3). Based on these estimates of incidence, the lifetime prevalence seems lower than expected, especially since the illness is usually chronic. This discrepancy may be due to two other facts about the disorder: some patients recover and there is a

Table 5.1 Point prevalence of schizophrenia

Study	Location	Prevalence per 1000
Brugger (1931)	Germany	2.4
Brugger (1933)	Germany	2.2
Klemperer (1933)	Germany	10.0
Strömgren (1935)	Denmark	3.3
Lemkao (1936)	USA	2.9
Roth and Luton (1938)	USA	1.7
Brugger (1938)	Germany	2.3
Lin (1946–1948)	China	2.1
Mayer-Gross (1948)	Scotland	4.2
Bremer (1951)	Norway	4.4
Böök (1953)	Sweden	9.5
Larson (1954)	Sweden	4.6
National Survey (1954)	Japan	2.3
Essen-Möller (1956)	Sweden	6.7
Yoo (1961)	Korea	3.8
Juel-Nielsen (1962)	Denmark	1.5
Ivanys (1963)	Czechoslovakia	1.7
Krasik (1965)	USSR	3.1
Hagnell (1966)	Sweden	4.5
Wing (1967)	England	4.4
	Scotland	2.5
	USA	7.0
Lin (1969)	Taiwan	1.4
Jayasundera (1969)	Ceylon	3.2
Kato (1969)	Japan	2.3
Dube (1970)	India	3.7
Roy (1970)	Canada	
	Indians	5.7
	Non-Indians	1.6
Crocetti (1971)	Yugoslavia	
	Rijeka	7.3
	Zagreb	4.2
Kulcar (1971)	Yugoslavia	
	Lubin	7.4
	Sinj-Trogir	2.9
Bash (1972)	Iran	2.1
Zharikov (1972)	USSR	5.1

(continued)

Table 5.1 Continued

Study	Location	Prevalence per 1000
Babigian (1975)	USA	4.7
Temkov (1975)	Bulgaria	2.8
Rotstein (1977)	USSR	3.8
Nielsen (1977)	Denmark	2.7
Ouspenskaya (1978)	USSR	5.3
Böök (1978)	Sweden	17.0
Lehtinen (1978)	Finland	15.0
Wijesinghe (1978)	Ceylon	5.6
Weissman (1980)	USA	4.0
Hafner (1980)	Germany	1.2
Walsh (1980)	Ireland	8.3
Rin (1982)	Taiwan	0.9
Sikanartey (1984)	Ghana	0.6
Meyers (1984)	USA	
	New Haven	11.0
	Baltimore	10.0
	St Louis	6.0
Von Korff (1985)	Baltimore	6.0
Hwu (1989)	Taiwan	2.4
Astrup (1989)	Norway	7.3
Bøjholm (1989)	Denmark	3.3
Lee (1990)	Korea	3.1
Stefánsson (1991)	Iceland	3.0
Youssef (1991)	Ireland	3.3
Chen (1993)	China	1.3
de Salvia (1993)	Italy	1.4
Kendler (1994)	Ireland	5.3
Jeffreys (1997)	UK	5.1
Myles-Worsley (1999)	Palau	19.9
Waldo (1999)	Micronesia	6.8
Kebede (1999)	Ethiopia	7.1
Nimgaonkar (2000)	Canada	1.2
Jablensky (2000)	Australia	4.5
Chan (2015)	China (urban)	8.3
	China (rural)	5.0
Binnbay (2016)	Turkey	3.6

Table 5.2 Lifetime prevalence of schizophrenia

Study	Country	Lifetime prevalence per 1000
Hagnell (1966)	Sweden	14.0
Brugger (1931)	Germany	3.8
Brugger (1933)	Germany	4.1
Klemperer (1933)	Germany	14.0
Brugger (1938)	Germany	3.6
Strömgren (1938)	Denmark	5.8
Ødegard (1946)	Norway	18.7
Fremming (1947)	Denmark	9.0
Böök (1953)	Sweden	26.6
Sjögren (1954)	Sweden	16.0
Helgason (1964)	Iceland	8.0
Helgason (1977)	Iceland	4.9
Böök (1978)	Sweden	24.8
Robins (1984)	USA	19.0
	New Haven	19.0
	Baltimore	16.0
	St Louis	10.0
Widerlov (1989)	Denmark	37.0
Hwu (1989)	Taiwan	2.6
Lehtinen (1990)	Finland	13.0
Youssef (1991)	Ireland	6.4
Bijl (1998)	The Netherlands	4.0
Thavichachart (2001)	Thailand	13.0
Binbay (2016)	Turkey	9.8

twofold increase in early death among people with schizophrenia relative to the general population.

The lifetime risk rates for schizophrenia are more variable across studies than the prevalence or incidence rates. This increased variability is probably due to methodological differences in how the rates are computed. The difference in the prevalence, incidence, and lifetime risk rates highlights the importance of using these terms correctly. As our discussion shows, the risk for developing schizophrenia over one's lifetime is much higher than either the incidence or prevalence of the disorder.

Table 5.3 Incidence of schizophrenia

Study	Country	Annual number of new cases per 1000
Ødegaard (1946)	Norway	0.24
Hollingshead (1958)	USA	0.30
Norris (1959)	UK	0.17
Jaco (1960)	USA	0.35
Dunham (1965)	USA	0.52
Warthen (1967)	USA	0.70
Adelstein (1968)	UK	0.26–0.35
Walsh (1969)	Ireland	0.46–0.57
Hafner (1970)	Germany	0.54
Lieberman (1974)	USSR	0.19–0.20
Hailey (1974)	UK	0.10–0.14
Babigian (1975)	USA	0.69
Nielsen (1976)	Denmark	0.20
Helgason (1977)	Iceland	0.27
Krupinski (1983)	Australia	0.18
Folnegovic (1990)	Croatia	0.22
Youssef (1991)	Ireland	0.16
Jablensky (1992)	Colombia	0.09
Folnegovic (1990)	Croatia	0.22
Jablensky (1992)	USA	0.12
Jablensky (1992)	USA	0.13
Jablensky (1992)	UK	0.19
Jablensky (1992)	Russia	0.15
Jablensky (1992)	Nigeria	0.11
Jablensky (1992)	Japan	0.16
Jablensky (1992)	Ireland	0.16
Jablensky (1992)	India	0.25
Jablensky (1992)	Denmark	0.13
Jablensky (1992)	Czech Republic	0.08
Nicole (1992)	Canada	0.20
McNaught (1997)	UK	0.21
Preti (2000)	Italy	0.88
Rajkumar (1993)	India	0.41
Mahy (1999)	Barbados	0.32
Hickling (1991)	Jamaica	0.24
Svedberg (2001)	Sweden	0.17
Hanoeman (2002)	Surinam	0.16
Tortelli (2015)	England	0.12

According to the latest figures from the World Health Organization (WHO), an estimated 21 million people worldwide are affected with schizophrenia at any point in time, and as many as 51 million will be affected at some point in their lifetime. While not a leading cause of death, schizophrenia is among the top ten conditions causing moderate to severe disability, with 16.7 million people at this level of disability globally. The majority of these (65%) were under the age of 60. Not surprisingly, countries defined by WHO to be low- or middle income (i.e., having a gross national income per capita <$10,066) had a disproportionate share (84%) of this group.

To provide a sense of the burden of this disease, the WHO has calculated a measure, called the disability-adjusted life year (DALY), which 'can be thought of as one lost year of 'healthy' life' due to death or disability. Using this metric, the low- and middle-income countries carry an even greater burden of this disease, accounting for 91% of the years of healthy life lost to schizophrenia.

6

Is schizophrenia inherited?

→ Key points

- Schizophrenia runs in families. The lifetime risk for the siblings and children of people with schizophrenia is anywhere between 4% and 14%, which is about ten times higher than the risk in the general population.

- Identical twins come from the same fertilized egg, whereas fraternal twins come from different eggs fertilized at the same time. Thus, identical twins are 100% similar genetically, whereas fraternal twins are 50% similar. If one twin has schizophrenia, the probability of the other twin also having schizophrenia is 53% for identical twins and 15% for fraternal twins. This finding shows that schizophrenia is not entirely a genetic disorder, but has a strong genetic component.

- Adoption studies show that schizophrenia risk is transmitted to the biological relatives of patients, not the adoptive relatives, which suggests that schizophrenia runs in families due to genes, not learning or bad parenting.

- Many risk genes for schizophrenia have been discovered, but most of the genes that cause the disorder are unknown.

We have known for some time, from family studies done in Europe in the first half of the 1900s, that schizophrenia runs in families. These studies found the risks for the parents, brothers, and sisters of people with schizophrenia to be between 4% and 14%—on average about ten times as high as that for the general population. For children of those with schizophrenia, the risk was 12%, nearly 15 times the general population risk. When both parents had schizophrenia, the risk increased to about 40%. The risk to uncles and aunts, nephews and nieces, grandchildren, and half-brothers or -sisters was roughly three times the risk in the general population. This risk was much lower than the risk to the relatives in the immediate family circle. On the whole, these pioneering studies showed that the closer the blood relationship of a person to an individual with schizophrenia, the higher the risk for the disorder (Figure 6.1).

Modern studies using more strict research methods and reliable definitions of schizophrenia also found the disorder to run in families. However, they find risk estimates that are a bit lower than those found in earlier studies. For example, in a large family study from Iowa, Tsuang and his team reported the risk of schizophrenia to brothers and sisters of individuals with schizophrenia

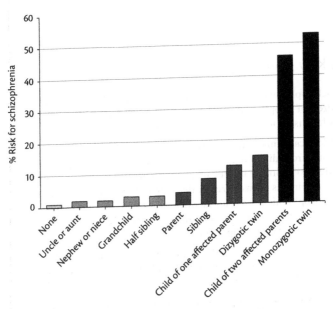

Relationship to individual with schizophrenia

Figure 6.1 Risk by Degree of Relatedness. The per cent risk for schizophrenia is plotted on the vertical axis, and the degree of relatedness to an individual with schizophrenia is plotted on the horizontal axis. Furthest to the left, the risk to someone in the general population with no known relationship to an individual with schizophrenia is the same as the prevalence of the disorder: about 1%. In the next four light-grey bars, we show the risk to second-degree relatives of an individual with schizophrenia (who share 25% of genes in common), which ranges from approximately 2% to 4%. In the next four dark-grey bars, we show the risk to first-degree relatives of an individual with schizophrenia (who share 50% of genes in common), which ranges from approximately 4% to 14%. In the last two black bars, we show the risk to first-degree relatives of an individual with schizophrenia (but here only those who share 100% of genes in common), which ranges from approximately 45% to 55%.

to be about 3%. This level of risk was five times greater than the risk to relatives of persons without schizophrenia. Other modern studies found similar results. Diagnostic practises seem to play a strong role in these different estimates. The early European studies usually used a fairly broad definition of the illness while the modern studies used a strict criterion-based diagnosis developed for use in research. Indeed, modern researchers have noted that their family risk figures for schizophrenia are similar to the figures obtained by the earlier European studies when atypical cases are included in the definition of schizophrenia. In other words, the level of risk that we can pin on a family history of schizophrenia depends on how broadly we define the disorder and whether or not we include atypical cases and spectrum disorders.

Although these family patterns suggest a hereditary part to schizophrenia, they could also be explained by causes in the environment shared within the family. Thus, some traits that run in families, such as eye colour, are determined by genes, but others, such as one's spoken language, are learned and not due to genes. To pull apart heredity and environment, we need data from twin and adoption studies.

Twin studies

There are two types of twins: monozygotic (or identical) and dizygotic (or fraternal). Identical twins come from one fertilized egg and thus they have the exact same sets of genes. Fraternal twins come from two different fertilized eggs and thus share only half their genes on average; they are like ordinary brothers and sisters except that they were conceived at the same time. Within a twin-pair, if both twins have schizophrenia, they are said to be concordant for schizophrenia; if one has schizophrenia and the other does not, they are called discordant.

If schizophrenia were due to genes only, the concordance rates for identical twins would be 100%, and the rate for fraternal twins would be 50%. However, even if the disorder were only partly genetic (and partly environmental), different rates of concordance in the two types of twin-pairs would be revealing. For example, if we see a much higher concordance rate for schizophrenia in identical twin-pairs than in fraternal twin-pairs, this points to at least some role for genes in the disorder. On the other hand, if schizophrenia were entirely due to the environment, there would be no difference in the concordance rates for identical and fraternal twin-pairs, since both types of twin-pairs have a common environment.

Putting together the results of twin studies from different parts of the world, we see concordance rates of about 53% for identical twin-pairs and 15% for fraternal twin-pairs. This finding shows that there must be a hereditary part to schizophrenia; in fact, a meta-analysis of twin studies estimates that 81% of the risk for schizophrenia is due to genes. The fact that the concordance rate for identical twin-pairs is not 100% shows that this is not simply a genetic disorder, but that environment plays a part as well.

The results from twin studies are clear enough, but such studies have been criticized because being raised as a twin may confuse self-identity, particularly in identical twin-pairs where one twin can easily be mistaken for the other. However, if confusion of self-identity leads to higher concordance rates of schizophrenia for identical twins, one would expect to find a higher risk for schizophrenia in people who are part of an identical-twin pair than in the general population. Because such higher rates have not been observed, we concluded that confusion of self-identity is not causing schizophrenia in twins.

Another explanation for the higher concordance rate in identical twin-pairs than fraternal twin-pairs is that they are exposed to more similar environmental risk factors. This hypothesis has been tested by looking at co-twins who were separated at birth and raised in different environments. A high concordance rate for identical twin-pairs reared apart would argue against the idea that sharing the same environmental risks leads to their higher concordance rate. More than half of such identical twin-pairs have been reported to be concordant for schizophrenia, thus further supporting the genetic explanation.

Despite the methodological limits of twin studies, on the whole they do give evidence for a strong hereditary piece in schizophrenia, but they also show that the environment plays some role too.

Adoption studies

More evidence for the role of heredity in schizophrenia comes from adoption studies. In the 1960s, pioneering adoption studies were carried out in the USA and Denmark. In the USA, Dr Leonard Heston examined 47 children in Oregon who had been separated within 3 days of birth from their biological mothers with schizophrenia. These children were raised by adoptive parents with whom they had no biological relationship. He also studied a comparison group of 50 individuals who had been adopted away from mothers who did not have schizophrenia. The idea behind the study was to see if children born to mothers with schizophrenia would have a higher chance of developing schizophrenia than children born to mothers who did not have the disorder. The beauty of this study design is that no member of either group had been exposed for very long to his or her own biological mother or to any other biological relative. If genes cause schizophrenia, then the biological children of mothers with schizophrenia should have a higher risk for schizophrenia regardless of who raised them. In contrast, if the parenting relationship (i.e., the environment) causes schizophrenia, then separating children from a parent with schizophrenia should prevent them from developing schizophrenia. Dr Heston's results were clear: five children of mothers with schizophrenia developed the disorder, but no cases of the illness were seen among the children of mothers without schizophrenia. This gave us convincing evidence for a hereditary piece in schizophrenia.

In Denmark, where excellent national and medical databases are kept, Dr Seymour Kety and his team from the US National Institute of Mental Health, along with Dr Fini Schulsinger from Denmark, carried out adoption studies of schizophrenia. In the Greater Copenhagen area a total of 5500 children were adopted away from their biological families between 1923 and 1947. Of these children, 33 who later developed schizophrenia were studied along with 33 comparison adoptees without the disorder. To avoid bias from their hypotheses, some members of the team studied the biological relatives of these adoptees without knowing if they belonged to a family with or without schizophrenia in it.

Drs Kety and Schulsinger found that 21% of the biological relatives of an individual with schizophrenia also developed schizophrenia or a related disorder, while a rate of only 11% was found in the biological relatives of the comparison adoptees without schizophrenia. They found no differences in rates of schizophrenia between the adoptive relatives of the adoptees with or without schizophrenia. The findings provided additional, strong evidence for the genetic basis of schizophrenia.

One component of the Danish study was similar to Dr Heston's American study. Children born into families affected by schizophrenia but raised by families without the illness were compared with children born to, and raised by, parents without schizophrenia. In line with the genetic theory of the disorder, schizophrenia and related disorders were found in 32% of the first group but only in 18% of the second group.

These adoption studies show that parents with schizophrenia transmit the risk towards the illness to their children even when these children are reared by parents without the disorder. These studies show that biological and genetic relationships impact the risk for schizophrenia. They also indicate that parenting does not cause schizophrenia. Fortunately, the Danish samples provided a direct test of whether or not being raised by a parent with schizophrenia could cause the disorder. This direct test was possible because the Danish sample included some persons who had been born to parents who did not have schizophrenia but were then raised by a parent with schizophrenia. If being reared by a parent with schizophrenia caused the disorder, then these persons should be more likely than average to suffer from the disorder. Contrary to this idea, the team found that rearing by a parent with schizophrenia did not cause schizophrenia in a child who was not genetically predisposed to the disorder.

Findings from adoption studies thus strengthen the case that heredity (not environment) is the chief reason that schizophrenia runs in families. However, these studies have some limitations. Although the American and Danish investigators tried to separate genetic and environmental factors, they could not succeed completely. Dr Kety pointed out that even though an adopted child had been separated from the mother soon after birth, the child had spent nine months in the mother's uterus and some time with her immediately after the birth. During that time, the mother could have transmitted to the foetus or young baby some non-genetic biological or psychosocial factor that might have contributed to the child's schizophrenia many years later.

What factor could cause such delayed effects? One candidate is a slow virus, which could lie dormant for years before being triggered by some later bio-logical and psychosocial conditions. If a mother carried such a virus, she could transmit it to her child while the child was in her uterus. No such slow virus has been discovered, but the data from family, twin, and adoption studies do not rule out the possibility that one might exist.

Fortunately, the Danish researchers could test whether or not *in utero* factors might have explained the results of their adoption studies. They studied a group of blood relatives who had not been exposed to the same uterine environment. These were half-brothers or half-sisters (from the father's side) of children who had been adopted away and later developed schizophrenia. These paternal half-siblings had the same father but different mothers. Dr Kety and his team found that 8 of 63 paternal half-siblings of adoptees with schizophrenia (12.7%) had the disorder compared with only 1 of 64 paternal half-siblings of adoptees without schizophrenia (1.6%). Because paternal half-siblings have different mothers, these results cannot be explained by *in utero* effects. Indeed, the fact that a higher rate of schizophrenia was found among these half-siblings from the father's side, than in the half-siblings of the comparison adoptees, gave the most solid evidence yet for the hereditary basis of schizophrenia.

The Danish adoption study results were later found again in another, provin-cial, Danish sample. Taken together—along with Heston's adoption study and others that came after—the Danish work drove a large scientific effort on under-standing how the heritable risk for schizophrenia passes through families.

The mechanism of genetic transmission

Although family, twin, and adoption studies show that schizophrenia is at least partly caused by genes, it has been surprisingly hard for scientists to find the mechanism of genetic transmission; that is, what specific genes are responsible, how they are passed on, and how they work together. There are several possi-bilities. At one extreme it may be that a problem in a single gene is the genetic cause of schizophrenia. At the other extreme, is the *Anna Karenina* scenario; as the Tolstoy novel began, 'All happy families are alike; each unhappy family is unhappy in its own way.' So it may be that each person with schizophrenia may have a 'personal aetiology' that is unique, whereby there are as many genetic causes and types of schizophrenia as there are people with schizophrenia. In between is a situation where many genes act in combination with one another, and with the environment, to cause the illness.

Our genes, and traits driven by those genes, are passed on according to biological laws. These laws have a mathematical description that predicts the pattern of illness in families. It is, therefore, possible to use family, twin, and adoption studies to test whether one, several, or very many genes are the cause of schizophrenia. Sadly, attempts to fit mathematical genetic models to schizophrenia family data have not given clear results. Some studies support the idea of a single responsible gene in some families, but most others find that many genes would be needed to explain the pattern of transmission seen in most families with schizophrenia.

Scientists studying diseases such as cystic fibrosis and Huntington's disease have shown that it is possible to find single genes that always cause illness. We call these *simple* or Mendelian disorders, so-named because they are inherited in the same predictable way as the traits of the pea plants studied by Gregor Mendel in the 1800s. The pattern of family transmission of these and many other disorders closely follows the laws of single-gene inheritance. In contrast, the exact mode of inheritance of schizophrenia is unknown and does not conform to the laws of inheritance for single-gene disorders. In such cases, we call the mode of inheritance *complex*. Modern methods of association analysis are well equipped to find the large number of genes that make even very small contributions to an individual's overall risk for a disorder, as long as those small effects are consistent and reliable across individuals (Figure 6.2).

Association studies

In the early part of the 2000s, laboratory technology improved to the point where we could directly test all parts of the genome for association with the disorder, using an approach called **genome-wide association scanning**, or GWAS.

The genome refers to all of the individual pieces of DNA that make us similar as a species but different as individuals. Our genome comprises some six billion 'bases' of DNA spread across 23 pairs of 'chromosomes'; one part of each pair of chromosomes is inherited from the mother and the other part is inherited from the father. Each variant of the DNA at a given spot, or 'locus', in the genome is called an allele, and the combination of two alleles (one from the mother and one from the father) at a given locus is called a genotype (Figure 6.3).

If a gene increases the risk for schizophrenia, this shows up as an increased number of risk versions or variants of the gene in individuals with schizophrenia

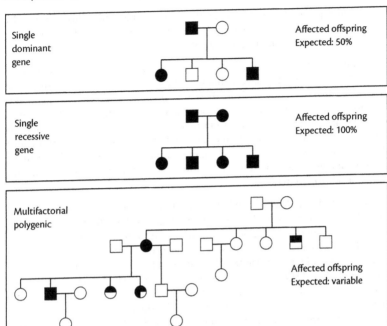

Figure 6.2 Mode of Genetic Transmission. Genes play a role in most human traits, including many diseases. There are a number of ways in which genes can cause or influence traits and diseases. In the case of a single 'dominant' gene that causes a disease (top panel), when one parent has a copy of the disease-causing gene (and the disease himself) and the other parent does not, each child has a 50:50 chance of either having or not having the same gene and disease as the affected parent. In the case of a single 'recessive' gene that causes a disease (middle panel), when both parents have the disease-causing gene (and the disease themselves), each child will also have the gene and the disease. In the case of a disease caused by the combined effects of many genes as well as environmental effects (called a 'multifactorial polygenic' mode of inheritance, bottom panel), a portion of the large number of disease-associated risk genes are passed on to all individuals in various combinations. The confluence of enough risk genes plus environmental factors in any given individual can be random, and lead to an unpredictable pattern of disease in the family. A family with many affected ancestors will have a higher probability than other families of having affected descendants, but even in heavily affected families, many individuals will be unaffected, or just partly affected. Similarly, the disease can emerge in descendants of other families even where there is not a strong family history of the disease. Most families affected by schizophrenia do not show a pattern of inheritance consistent with either a dominant or recessive gene, but rather a multifactorial polygenic pattern. Note: squares represent males, circles represent females; black shading indicates presence of a disease, white shading indicates absence of a disease, and partial shading indicates a partial form of the disorder, such as a spectrum disorder; older generations are at the top of each pedigree.

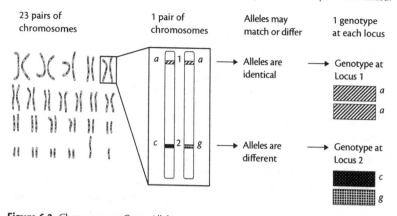

Figure 6.3 Chromosome, Gene, Allele.
Clip art image reproduced under the terms of the Creative Commons Attribution 3.0 Unported license (CC BY 3.0), https://creativecommons.org/licenses/by/3.0/ from Smart Servier Medical Art, https://smart.servier.com/

compared to individuals without schizophrenia. This type of study is usually done by comparing a large group of biologically unrelated people with schizophrenia against a separate group of people without schizophrenia, but who are similar in all other regards to those with schizophrenia. In such a 'case–control association study', we count the number of each type of variant of a gene found in those with schizophrenia and compare these counts with those seen in people without schizophrenia. A simple statistical test determines if any genetic variant is reliably more common in individuals with schizophrenia. If we find such a difference, we refer to the variant that is more common among the affected individuals as a risk variant. In the context of the family, association studies look for a higher rate of individuals with schizophrenia receiving the risk variant of the gene from his or her parent, even when both the risk and normal variants of the gene were present in the parents and had an equal chance of being inherited.

Many scientists have used the GWAS approach to find risk genes for schizophrenia. Since the results of GWAS are very simple to interpret, it is also easy for different groups of scientists to put their results together to get a more accurate picture of the genetic reality of schizophrenia. The world's largest group of schizophrenia genetics researchers, to which we also belong, is called the Psychiatric Genomics Consortium. We and dozens of other groups from around the world have put our GWAS results together by meta-analysis to come up with our best estimates of the genetic variants that most strongly and reliably increase risk for the disorder. After decades of hard work, it is rewarding to have finally found a large number (~250) of places in the genome where individual differences are tied to risk for the disorder. These sites are spread widely across our 23 pairs of chromosomes, so there is not just one or a few concentrated areas in our DNA where risk genes lie. Although finding these 250 risk regions marks a dramatic turning point in our understanding of the disorder, they only tell us that the region discovered harbours a piece of DNA that increases the risk for schizophrenia; it does not pinpoint its exact location. Thus, identification of risk regions by GWAS is only the first crucial step on a long path toward understanding the genetic causes of schizophrenia, and using that knowledge to develop better diagnostic tests or improved treatments.

When we put together a list of the strongest risk genes for schizophrenia, we can explain a good portion of the heritable risk for the disorder (but recall that schizophrenia is not completely inherited; the environment also plays a role that GWAS cannot identify). Thus, twin studies tell us that about 60–85% of the risk for schizophrenia is inherited, and GWAS tells us that approximately 20% of risk has been found and attached to the top genes. Each single gene variant typically increases an individual's risk of schizophrenia by about 10% or less relative to baseline risk. So if the overall population risk for schizophrenia is approximately 1%, having any given risk–gene variant may bump that risk only to 1.1%. On its own, no single risk–gene variant is enough to cause schizophrenia, and in fact, each of us is carrying many risk variants for the disorder. It is only in combination with many other risk variants, and environmental risk factors that these genes bring about the disorder.

Scientists are still working hard to figure out why there is such a large gap between the 60–85% of schizophrenia risk that is heritable and the 20% of risk that has been found for the top genes. In all likelihood, the size of this 'missing heritability' can be reduced by finding interactions between genes, and interactions of genes with environmental factors. Beyond these approaches, it also seems likely that some of the risk for schizophrenia comes not from small changes to the genome sequence such as those pinpointed by GWAS, but from large structural changes to the DNA.

Copy-number variation

Ironically, the development of technology to perform GWAS, which was meant to simplify the approach to finding genetic risk factors for schizophrenia, has in fact only shed light on just how complex the human genome is and how a variety of different genetic mechanisms may be operating in this illness. One such complexity has been the discovery of large insertions or deletions of DNA known as copy-number variations, or CNVs. CNVs are rare but are more common in people with the disorder than in those without. Also, the exact regions of the genome that are inserted or deleted in schizophrenia differ widely among affected individuals, suggesting that there are, again, variable paths from genomic variation to disorder. Apart from being quite rare, these large insertions and deletions do not, on their own, account for a large amount of risk in the population. However, for individuals who have, for example, a deletion of a large part of their 22nd chromosome or duplication of a large part of their 16th chromosome, their risk is dramatically increased (anywhere from two to ten times higher than the risk to the general population). The discovery of CNVs has one big advantage over the discovery of risk regions by GWAS. A CNV discovery tells us exactly what piece of DNA is changed in persons with schizophrenia, which is helpful for understanding the biology of the disorder. For GWAS regions, more work is needed to be as certain of the biological significance of the finding.

The biology of schizophrenia-risk genes

Although it is too soon to say that GWAS has 'solved' the genetic and biological riddle of schizophrenia, it has begun to give us clues about the biological features that contribute to the disorder. If we look at the strongest risk genes discovered by GWAS, they are not random with regard to their biological functions. The single strongest risk region for schizophrenia is on chromosome 6 within a section of that chromosome called the major histocompatibility complex (**MHC**). The MHC contains many genes that tell our body how to identify and protect itself from foreign molecules, such as viruses. Studies of the MHC suggest that a gene called C4A is the schizophrenia risk gene that accounts for the GWAS finding. C4A encodes the complement 4A protein.

It has been surprising that the strongest biological system associated with genetic risk for schizophrenia is the immune system, and this is changing our understanding of what immune system genes do. Aside from coordinating immune system responses, for example, C4A has recently been found to play a role in the way brain cells, or neurons, develop in early life, and how they mature. Apart from the immune system and neuron development, risk genes for schizophrenia also impact the biology of dopamine neurons, which is important because all medications that help with the positive symptoms of schizophrenia also interact with dopamine neurons. In addition, schizophrenia-risk genes impact a process called cell adhesion, which governs how cells make connections with other cells. Furthermore, schizophrenia-risk genes often are involved in calcium transport, a process by which this vital element is moved in and out of cells to regulate their electrical energy. So although the genes for schizophrenia are distributed widely across the genome, they have common threads at the level of biology. They are especially concentrated in areas such as immunity, cell adhesion and 'signalling' or communication between cells, and cellular activation.

Effects of schizophrenia-risk genes on other disorders

Like family and twin studies before them, GWAS studies have shown a clear heritable contribution to schizophrenia. Moreover, like those family and twin studies, GWAS also shows that schizophrenia does not simply increase the risk for schizophrenia in families; it also increases the risk for other related disorders, such as schizophrenia spectrum disorders, but also mood disorders like bipolar disorder and major depressive disorder. At the level of CNVs, however, schizophrenia has much more in common with autism spectrum disorders and with intellectual disability. In fact, recent research shows that virtually every large duplication or deletion that increases the risk for an autism spectrum disorder or intellectual disability also increases the risk for schizophrenia, and vice versa.

Genetic heterogeneity

The wide variety of genetic results for schizophrenia that have emerged in the past 15 years sometimes gives scientists pause, as it abolishes all hope that there will be a single, simple explanation for the disorder. Instead, the data show that many cases of schizophrenia are due to individual or combinations of rare variants that are exclusive to a small number of families or individuals. To further complicate matters, some of these variants are not inherited; they are acquired *de novo* during one's lifetime due to new mutations that introduce new alleles. In the best-case scenario (which we have already ruled out), schizophrenia would be caused by one factor, either genetic or environmental. This would simplify diagnosis and dictate a straightforward intervention to offset that genetic (or environmental) effect. In the worst case scenario (the *Anna Karenina* scenario), each affected individual has his or her own constellation of risk factors, which makes diagnosis, treatment, and even research much more difficult. We have long assumed that the true scenario lies between these two extremes, but the recent data from GWAS and other genetic studies suggest that the answer may lie closer to the more heterogeneous and complex scenario. These leads, and others generated from GWAS, are now a top research priority and are being vigorously pursued.

Collectively, the studies to date show that GWAS can find genes that increase the risk for schizophrenia and implicate new biological pathways involved in the disorder. Yet, as described above, these studies have limitations that may prevent us from detecting all of the associated genes or identifying the truly responsible variation at each site in the genome. New technologies will need to be brought to bear on schizophrenia to hasten the rate of risk-gene discovery. Direct DNA sequencing, which 15 years ago could only be accomplished on one individual's genome at the cost of over one million dollars, has recently become feasible. In fact, even now, the most advanced studies of the disorder are using whole-genome sequencing to identify risk-associated variants. Soon, whole-genome data on affected individuals will be available in sufficient numbers and from enough groups of scientists to enable the same sort of data-sharing that was done for GWAS data. This will undoubtedly usher in discoveries that complement those from GWAS to paint a more complete picture of the risk genes for the disorder and to find true causal variation that can be acted upon.

Epigenetics

We refer to how the environment modifies the output of the genome as 'epigenetic' effects. These effects occur throughout the human genome and have a huge impact on the expression of genes. Epigenetic effects do not change the sequence of the DNA or the type of protein that is built by the DNA. Instead, they can turn genes 'on' and 'off' (like a light switch) or regulate how much protein is produced by the gene (like a light dimmer). In so doing, they can direct how much or how little of a protein is made.

We are now seeing some concrete examples where genetic variants that usually increase the risk for schizophrenia may be made more or less powerful depending on the epigenetic modifications affecting that gene. We are just beginning to map normal and schizophrenia-associated epigenetic modifications in the genome, so it will be some time before we can develop a decent understanding of the true impact of epigenetics on schizophrenia risk, its underlying biology, and potentially its treatment. We anticipate that epigenetics may ultimately provide a means for better predicting the risk for the disorder in conjunction with genetic variant data, understanding the ways the environment modifies the risk for schizophrenia, and perhaps designing novel avenues for therapeutic intervention.

The identification of numerous risk genes of varying effect on the risk towards schizophrenia may someday make it possible to create a genetic risk profile that will be predictive of future onsets of the disorder. Such a genetic risk profile may also find use in genetic counselling settings to help potential parents understand the risk of schizophrenia to their unborn child and to make informed decisions based on this information. Most relevant for the treatment of schizophrenia, several genes have also been found to influence the outcome of medication treatments. As the relationships between these genes and aspects of the favourable or unfavourable response to medications become further clarified, these too may have use in the clinic in the development of genetically tailored, personalized medication management of schizophrenia. We must emphasize, however, that such uses of genetic data are not possible at this time and may not be possible for some time.

7

How does the environment influence schizophrenia?

> ## ⊙ Key points
>
> ◆ Some environmental factors contribute to the risk for schizophrenia, while others change the symptoms of schizophrenia in individuals with the disorder.
>
> ◆ The term 'schizophrenogenic' was applied to mothers whose method of upbringing for their child was once thought to cause schizophrenia. Research shows that this idea is wrong.
>
> ◆ Social selection occurs when a geographic region either draws or deters individuals with schizophrenia due to the way of life there.
>
> ◆ The downward drift hypothesis states that individuals with schizophrenia who cannot perform in a job or function well in daily life will 'drift downward' in social class. In support of this hypothesis, researchers found that individuals with schizophrenia were of a lower socioeconomic class than their parents were at their age.
>
> ◆ Sporadic cases of schizophrenia are those without a family history of the disorder. These individuals are more likely to have brain abnormalities or atrophy and are more likely to have had birth complications.
>
> ◆ Stressful life events are often present when schizophrenia symptoms emerge.

Although there is very strong evidence for a genetic piece to schizophrenia, the lack of full concordance between identical twins shows that the environment also plays a role. We define an 'environmental risk factor' as any event that is not due to genes, specifically the individual differences in the DNA sequence.

These events may be biological (e.g., head injuries, viral infections), psychological (e.g., disrupted family relationships), or social (e.g., poverty).

Over the past few decades, scientists have found evidence for environmental risk factors in at least some cases of schizophrenia. Before reviewing this research, we must make an important distinction: some environmental factors may *cause* or contribute to schizophrenia while others *modify* or change the illness in someone who is already sick. In this book we use the term 'cause' to refer to any factor that can produce the illness or increase the chance of illness in someone who has not yet been affected by schizophrenia. This cause does not have to be either necessary or sufficient. This means that other causes may exist that also produce the illness, and that any given cause may need to interact with other causes for the disorder to occur. We use the term 'modifier' to refer to anything that changes the symptoms of the illness in someone who is already affected. As we discuss in a later chapter, knowing modifiers can help with the treatment of the disorder. However, they should not be confused with causes.

Do environmental risk factors cause schizophrenia?

Scientists who study schizophrenia and other psychiatric disorders have long ago abandoned the 'nature–nurture' controversy. In the past, many philosophers and scientists had taken one of two extreme positions. Some believed that psychiatric illness was only caused by innate or genetic factors; others felt that mental illness was the sole product of adverse environmental events. Today, we know that the question 'genes *or* environment?' is too simplistic. As Dr Paul Meehl realized several decades ago, the better question is much more complex: 'What group of environmental risk factors work together with which genes to produce schizophrenia?'

Before discussing specific environmental risk factors that may cause schizophrenia we should clarify why we believe that the study of such factors is essential. First, twin studies of schizophrenia show that the genetically identical co-twins of people with schizophrenia develop schizophrenia only 50% of the time. This is remarkable. When the co-twin of an individual with schizophrenia does not also have the disorder, this means that the schizophrenia-risk genes *require* an environmental event to trigger the genetic risk for the disorder. Twin studies show that, without a doubt, people can carry schizophrenia-risk genes without ever getting sick with the illness. This provides a strong rationale for the study of environmental events as risk factors for the disorder.

A second reason to study environmental risk factors is that they may be easier to change than genetic factors, and thus could be useful for treatment planning. Many environmental factors can be modified. For example, if specific diets or exposures caused schizophrenia, then public programmes or home-based therapies could be built with the goal of preventing the illness. Creating such treatments is the long-term goal of some scientists who study environmental risk factors.

Family relationships

In the mid-1900s, the mental health professions were dominated by theorists, scientists, and clinicians who thought that most mental illness was caused by events that interrupted, delayed, or otherwise disrupted psychological development. Since the family environment strongly impacts psychological well-being, it seemed wise to focus on family relationships as a potential cause of schizophrenia. Thus, theories of a role of the family in causing schizophrenia came from the observations made by clinicians.

Unfortunately, many of these theories were presented as fact without any scientific evidence. We hope in this chapter to show the advantage of rigorous scientific facts over myths, old wives' tales, and misunderstandings based on guesses and opinions. We start by discussing some old hypotheses that have now been discredited, but whose legacy can still be felt in current attitudes and stigmas about schizophrenia. It is sad to say that, before these theories had been shown to be false, many relatives, especially mothers, of individuals with schizophrenia had been told that their method of child-rearing caused the illness. This was a terrible burden to bear. We can only hope that most of these people have since learned the truth about these theories.

Schizophrenogenic mothers

At one time, many mental health clinicians and even researchers believed that personality traits of mothers caused schizophrenia in their children. These mothers were labelled 'schizophrenogenic' to indicate that they caused schizophrenia. The rationale for this theory was the belief—not fact—that mothers of individuals with schizophrenia tended to be overprotective, hostile, and unable to understand their children's feelings. These abnormal attitudes were thought to *create* schizophrenia symptoms and behaviours in their children.

However, this argument did not take into account the possibility that the mother's attitudes might develop *as a consequence* of having a child with schizophrenia. Even if it could be shown that the mother had such traits before the onset of her child's schizophrenia, it is possible that unusual characteristics of the at-risk child might have brought out such attitudes. There is also another possibility. The mothers of individuals with schizophrenia may have passed schizophrenia susceptibility genes to their child. Recall that many people who carry genetic risk factors for schizophrenia will not develop schizophrenia. They may have a personality disorder or may be completely normal. It is possible that the genetic contributors to schizophrenia may be expressed in traits such as overprotectiveness or hostility. Thus, any so-called schizophrenogenic traits might also be caused by the genetic causes of schizophrenia. We do not know why many clinicians embraced the theory of the schizophrenogenic mother, but studies have shown that the way in which mothers (or fathers) rear their children does not cause (or prevent) schizophrenia.

Double-bind theory

Mothers or mothers-to-be reading this book may wonder whether fathers of individuals with schizophrenia have also been studied. If the parent–child relationship is important, then surely the father's personality should also be considered. And, in fact, fathers were included in another theory that implicated a particular type of faulty communication, which could involve the mother or the father. In this 'double-bind' communication, the child is repeatedly exposed to opposing messages. For example, the parent might tell the child that she may go out but, at the same time, forbid her to do so with a contradictory gesture. The parent's verbal message requires one response, whereas that parent's deeper message requires the opposite.

The double-bind theory of schizophrenia appeared to explain some of the behaviour of individuals with schizophrenia. Such communication had the potential to make them withdraw into a fantasy world. Also, it seemed to encourage, if not teach, irrational behaviour. However, the double-bind theory grew out of a small number of clinical observations of the relationship between people with schizophrenia and their parents. At first sight both logical and plausible, it was widely applied to the treatment of schizophrenia, until conclusive evidence from well-designed experiments made it suspect. Today, it is no longer commonly believed and applied in the treatment of schizophrenia.

Parents' marital relationship

Another environmental hypothesis focused on the possibility that an abnormal relationship between mothers and fathers caused schizophrenia in their children. The basic idea here was that children observing the inappropriate behaviour of their parents would learn to respond with irrational, psychotic behaviour. Two kinds of abnormal marital relationships were characterized. The first was called the 'skewed' relationship. This occurred when one parent always gave way to the abnormal parent who then dominated the family. This relationship was thought to be often found among parents of males with schizophrenia. The mother tended to be dominant and the father passive. Consequently, the mother, unable to find emotional satisfaction from the father, turned to her son instead.

The other abnormal marital relationship was called 'marital schism'. In these relationships, the parents were in chronic conflict. Each ignored their mutual needs to pursue their own separate goals. In the process, each competed for the child's support. Proponents of this hypothesis said that marital schism was common between the parents of females with schizophrenia.

The ideas of marital skew and marital schism originated from interviews with a small number of families having a child with schizophrenia. However, later studies have shown that these two abnormal marital relationships are also found very often in families without any children with schizophrenia. There is no reason to believe that such relationships are specific to the parents of individuals with schizophrenia. Thus, we can conclude that abnormal parental marital relationships do not cause schizophrenia.

Disordered family communication

About 40 years ago, a study at the US National Institute of Mental Health set out to determine if disordered family communication caused schizophrenia. In a series of controlled experiments, patterns of family interaction were studied using taped interviews and psychological tests. The results, based on intensive studies of four families each having a child with schizophrenia, revealed that parents of individuals with schizophrenia displayed two types of disordered communication: the first was 'amorphous' thinking. It consisted of vague ideas without clear thinking. The second was 'fragmented' thinking, which described thoughts that were disjointed from one another. Here, the basic ideas expressed by the parents were clear, but the links between ideas were weak.

These two styles of communication were not restricted to one parent but were assumed to be characteristics of the family as a whole. The researchers theorized that these types of communication deviance influenced the cognitive development of the children. Consequently, the various kinds of thought disorder seen in schizophrenia were said to be a direct result of 'amorphous' and 'fragmented' family communications.

To test this hypothesis, scientists tested three parent groups based on the diagnoses of their children with schizophrenia, neurosis (relatively minor mental illness), or no mental disorder. Seventy-eight per cent of the parental pairs were classified correctly according to the diagnostic group of their children. It was found that the fathers of individuals with schizophrenia were more likely to be abnormal than the fathers of neurotic patients or normal comparison subjects, but no such difference was found between the mothers of the individuals with schizophrenia or neurosis.

An attempt to reproduce these findings at the University of London's Institute of Psychiatry produced different results. Using the same scoring system, the British investigators compared the parents of individuals with schizophrenia or neurosis. Although this study reproduced the finding about fathers, the characteristic differences between the fathers were less impressive than in the American study. This was probably because the British and American samples differed in their definitions of schizophrenia. In fact, whereas the British patients had positive schizophrenia symptoms of delusions and hallucinations, the American patients had more negative symptoms along with evidence of chronic personality disorganization.

It is possible that a genetic component in the style of communication may have affected the outcome. As stressed before, the interaction of genes and environment cannot be ignored in any family study. It is still uncertain whether disordered family communication is specific to schizophrenia or whether it could be found in a wide variety of mental illnesses. It is also likely that any abnormal communication observed among the parents is influenced by the same genes that confer risk for schizophrenia itself. Many of these parents may have had schizotypal personality disorder or other, mild manifestations of schizophrenia genes. However, if there is a causal relationship between abnormal communication and schizophrenia in offspring, improvements in family communication should prevent schizophrenia, and we know of no concrete evidence supporting this prediction. As such, we do not consider disordered communication in the family to be a cause of schizophrenia.

Children at risk for schizophrenia

Most of the family studies described so far were based on observations made after the affected individuals developed schizophrenia. Unfortunately, it is often difficult for patients and their families to remember accurately events that took place before the onset of schizophrenia. Another possible source of inaccuracy exists in these studies: abnormal characteristics in the parents could represent the response of the parents to the abnormal behaviour of their children. To eliminate these shortcomings, one would need to study children from birth to the time when some of them develop schizophrenia, recording all the characteristics of the children and the families. When one of the children in the study develops schizophrenia, the noteworthy characteristics of his family could be identified.

The lifetime risk for schizophrenia is about 1%. Thus, if 100 children were selected at birth for such a study, only one of them would have schizophrenia after 40 years of observations. To obtain 100 individuals with schizophrenia for study, we would need to follow 10,000 children from birth to the age of 40. Such a study, though ideal, is clearly impractical. One way to reduce the number of children for the study would be to select children with a high risk of developing schizophrenia. The best way to create such a sample is to study children of parents who, themselves, have schizophrenia. Since the lifetime risk of schizophrenia is about ten times higher in such children, the number of children under observation could be reduced by one-tenth. This strategy has been used to study biological aspects of schizophrenia but is unsuitable for the study of parental attitudes and family interaction because the selected children are already genetically predisposed to schizophrenia. It is therefore very difficult to separate the environmental and genetic components. Moreover, although the size of the sample can be reduced by studying only high-risk children and their families, the need for long-term follow-up makes such studies very time-consuming and expensive. It is sometimes possible, however, to use existing records from child guidance clinics and schools.

Studies based on such records, written long before the onset of schizophrenia, have shown that the parents of children who later go on to develop schizophrenia, particularly mothers, have more often been in conflict with their children, and demonstrated more signs of overconcern and protectiveness, than the parents of unaffected children. These parental abnormalities, however, cannot be regarded as evidence for a psychosocial theory of the cause of schizophrenia, unless genetic influences and the psychological reaction of the parents to the child's abnormal behaviour before the onset of schizophrenia can be ruled out. Studies of adoptive parents of individuals with schizophrenia have been designed specifically to separate the environmental and genetic influences of parental abnormalities on their children. As we reviewed earlier, adoption studies have found that schizophrenia is due more to genetic than to environmental transmission; no convincing evidence exists to support a direct link between parental rearing and the development of schizophrenia. On the contrary, adoption studies suggest that there is no causal relationship between rearing factors and schizophrenia.

Most notably, adoption studies have found an increased risk for schizophrenia among children born to mothers with schizophrenia and raised by persons without a history of psychiatric disorder. On the other hand, children born to non-mentally ill parents but raised by adoptive parents with severe mental illness did not show an increased rate of schizophrenia or associated disorders. These studies strongly indicate that rearing factors are not crucial to the development of schizophrenia.

Social environment

The studies of prevalence and incidence we discussed in previous chapters show that schizophrenia occurs around the world. It is not limited by geographic region, political system, economic system, or culture. However, the frequency of schizophrenia varies according to sociocultural background. Two extremes of the prevalence rate for schizophrenia were reported from a small community in northern Sweden on the one hand, and the Hutterites of North America on the other: the prevalence was 10.8 per 1000 in the former and 1.1 per 1000 in the latter. Such differences in prevalence between cultures led some researchers to hypothesize that sociocultural aspects of the environment might cause schizophrenia. In contrast, others argued that these differences were due to **social selection**. Social selection occurs when social or cultural characteristics of a region make it more or less likely that the mentally ill will move to or away from it. When this occurs, the culture of the community does not cause the illness; it merely makes it more or less likely that the affected individual will want to, or can, live there.

The Hutterites are a North American Anabaptist religious sect. They live austere and pious lives in a close-knit farming community. The probable explanation for the low prevalence of schizophrenia among the Hutterites is that those with schizophrenia-like traits would have moved out of such communities due to the high levels of social interaction expected by their peers. In north Sweden, the lifetime risk of schizophrenia was three times as high as in other Scandinavian areas. The climate in north Sweden is severe, and the people live extremely isolated lives. Such an environment might be appealing to individuals with schizophrenia. Also, people who do not have schizophrenia may not tolerate such extreme social isolation. They would tend to move away, leaving behind those who were genetically predisposed to schizophrenia and more tolerant of extreme social isolation. A high frequency of cousin marriages was also found in this isolated area; such marriages within a population which already carried genes for schizophrenia would have further increased the high risk of schizophrenia in this community.

Socioeconomic status

Epidemiological studies have taken a careful look at the relationship between socioeconomic status and mental illness. People living in the lower social classes are subjected to many disadvantages. Poverty, malnutrition, poor prenatal care of mothers, poor medical care, and chaotic family situations are a few examples of circumstances that could adversely affect mental health. It is reasonable to suggest that such factors will have a negative impact on the development of children, leading to an increased risk for schizophrenia. Researchers were not surprised when they found higher admission rates for schizophrenia among inner-city, low social class dwellers, in both Europe and America. According to a meta-analysis of several studies, living in the city raises the risk of schizophrenia more than twofold compared to living in the country. From these findings, some concluded that the social disorganization, economic deprivation, poor health, and limited educational opportunities among inner-city dwellers caused schizophrenia in predisposed persons. This raised a key question: 'Does low social class cause schizophrenia or does schizophrenia cause low social class?' It soon became apparent that both possibilities were equally likely. As we have described in previous chapters, schizophrenia leads to massive changes in perceptions, thinking, and social behaviour. Since many affected individuals cannot function well in school or on the job, they can 'drift downward' to the lower social classes. So, again, researchers faced the question of social causation versus social selection.

To examine the **downward drift** hypothesis, epidemiologists performed a simple test. If downward drift did not occur, then individuals with schizophrenia should have the same socioeconomic status that their parents did at the same age. However, studies showed that individuals with schizophrenia were more likely than unaffected comparison subjects to have a lower social status than their parents. Also, studies found that the fathers of individuals with schizophrenia did not differ in social class from the fathers of people without schizophrenia. Thus, individuals with schizophrenia are not exposed to the adversities of lower-class life more than individuals without the disorder.

A study by Dr Bruce Dohrenwend provided additional evidence that low social class does not cause schizophrenia. Dr Dohrenwend and his team noted that the study of disadvantaged ethnic groups could clarify this issue because, to some extent, their presence in the lower social classes is due to discrimination, not to lack of ability to achieve. He reasoned that if social adversity caused schizophrenia, and since discrimination is a form of social adversity, then minorities should be at *greater* risk for schizophrenia compared with non-minorities. Moreover, this increased risk for schizophrenia should be evident in all social classes. In contrast, if schizophrenia causes a downward drift in social class, then in the lower social classes, minorities should have a *lower* risk for schizophrenia. This prediction is based on the following reasoning. Because of discrimination, many members of minority groups who are psychiatrically healthy and capable of achievement will not move up in social class. If this is true, then their presence in the lower social classes should *decrease* the rate of schizophrenia in lower social-class minorities. In contrast, since non-minority individuals with schizophrenia would drift downward, this should *increase* the rate of schizophrenia in non-minority persons in the lower classes.

The results of this study supported the downward drift hypothesis. Most notable in this regard was the risk for schizophrenia among men in the lower social classes. This risk was 4% among the ethnically advantaged and 2% among the disadvantaged.

These findings, taken together with previous studies, suggest that schizophrenia causes patients to have a lower social class than they would have if they had not become ill. This is consistent with the fact that schizophrenia makes it very difficult for patients to deal effectively in social or occupational situations. Their social and occupational impairments make it likely that they will not achieve the high levels of economic and educational success required to move out of the lower social strata. Therefore, we and others have concluded that low socioeconomic status is a consequence, rather than a cause, of schizophrenia.

Schizophrenia as a symptom of a sick society

A minority of mental health professionals argue that schizophrenia is symptomatic of a sick society. From this viewpoint, schizophrenia is a means of coping with the unreasonable social forces exerted upon the affected individual. This social theory does not posit that low social class causes schizophrenia but rather that all social classes are at risk for the illness.

Surprisingly, the advocates of this hypothesis claim that the emergence of schizophrenia is a 'therapeutic experience'; the goal of therapy is to help guide the patient through this experience, not to stop it. These therapists believe that the pressures of our ailing society are exerted through the family and that one member of the family is singled out to bear the burden. 'Schizophrenia' is thought of as a label attached to this person as a result of the social process. Extreme followers of this theory regard the individual with schizophrenia as a person struggling to achieve freedom from the demands of his parents; by showing the signs of schizophrenia, he achieves his autonomy.

Since the psychotic symptoms of schizophrenia are seen as helpful to the patient, any treatment designed to cut short episodes of schizophrenia is, accordingly, thought to be antitherapeutic. Since the disturbed family relationship is the source of schizophrenia symptoms, treatment should not only involve the family but also aim at forming a special kind of corrective relationship between patient and therapist. Although some laypeople and professional workers accept this view of schizophrenia, it is not supported by scientific evidence.

Biological environmental risk factors

During the past five decades, scientists have moved away from studying family relationships and the social environment as primary causes of schizophrenia. Such theories failed to withstand the rigors of scientific testing, which led many to study environmental events that have biological significance for the developing human brain instead. At this point, the reader must understand that these events are called 'biological' as opposed to 'psychological' or 'social' because they are known to disturb biological functioning. Thus, we refer to factors such as social class and family relationships as non-biological because their impacts on biological functioning are unclear. In contrast, it is fairly easy to see how physical events like head injury or viral infection lead to brain damage. The biological implications of these latter events are straightforward. Thus, the distinction between biological and non-biological factors reflects our state of knowledge (or lack of it) regarding how events impact human biology. We can easily envision a day when the biological implications of psychological and social stresses are so well understood that the distinction we draw today between biological and non-biological events will no longer be needed.

Pregnancy and delivery complications

Any event that affects the fetus in the mother's womb *before* birth is classified as a prenatal event. These include physical trauma, malnutrition, infection, and intoxication. Perinatal events are those that occur *at* the time of birth. Examples are physical injury, lack of oxygen, infection, and bleeding. Events occurring *after* birth, whether biological or psychosocial, are called postnatal. When postnatal events occur close to the time of birth they are included with pre- and perinatal events under the term 'pregnancy and delivery complications', or **PDCs** for short.

Many studies have found increased rates of PDCs in the births of children who eventually developed schizophrenia. For example, individuals with schizophrenia are more likely to have been born prematurely and to have had relatively low birth weights. Other types of PDCs have also been found. What has puzzled researchers is that the association between PDCs and schizophrenia is not strong. Although individuals with schizophrenia are more likely to have had PDCs, these were fairly common in the general population. As a result, the great majority of babies who experienced the PDCs did not develop schizophrenia.

When researchers considered the PDC study results in combination with those of genetic studies, a simple, yet powerful hypothesis emerged. It appeared likely that the effect of PDCs was to activate the genetic predisposition to schizophrenia. They reasoned that the individual with schizophrenia inherits a liability or predisposition to develop schizophrenia. However, an environmental event is needed to trigger the predisposition. This is sometimes called the 'diathesis–stress' theory of schizophrenia because it requires both a genetic predisposition (diathesis) and an adverse environmental event (stress) for an individual to develop schizophrenia.

Dr Sarnoff Mednick found strong support for the diathesis–stress theory in a study of children born to mothers with schizophrenia. This study first showed that these 'high-risk' children were not more likely than other children to have PDCs. Thus, the presence of schizophrenia in the mother does not predict a more complicated birth for the child. This means that the genetic predisposition (having a mother with schizophrenia) is not confounded with the environmental stress (the PDCs). Dr Mednick and his team found that, *among* the group of high-risk children, PDCs were predictive of subsequent psychiatric abnormalities including schizophrenia. They also found that those children with the least complicated births were more likely to have 'borderline schizophrenia.' This refers to a syndrome that resembles schizophrenia in a very mild form. In today's diagnostic language we would say that they have schizotypal personality disorder. Overall, the results of this series of studies suggested that children with the genetic predisposition to schizophrenia were more likely to develop schizophrenia if they had PDCs.

The findings of Dr Mednick's group are intriguing, but, like many findings in schizophrenia, the final truth is likely to be more complex. There is general agreement that PDCs predict later schizophrenia and measurable brain abnormalities. Thus, it seems clear that PDCs have a certain biological impact. However, not all family studies support the idea that PDCs interact with a genetic predisposition to produce schizophrenia. Others have raised the possibility that PDCs cause a non-genetic form of schizophrenia. This alternative theory suggests that PDCs can cause schizophrenia in people who do not have the genetic predisposition. In support of this, several studies found more PDCs among patients without a family history of schizophrenia compared with patients with a family history. However, other studies find no difference. These findings highlight the complexity of the causal chain of events leading to schizophrenia. It seems likely that PDCs either add to the causal effects of genes or trigger these effects. In rare cases, they may act alone to cause a non-genetic form of schizophrenia.

The viral hypothesis

Most of us are familiar with viruses. These organisms, which cannot be seen without specialized microscopes, have made all of us ill at one time or another with mild colds, the flu, or digestive problems. We also know, from major epidemics such as AIDS, Ebola, and influenza, that viruses can be very dangerous. This tells us that viruses can have a wide range of effects, from mild discomfort to death. Thus, the reader will not be surprised by speculation that a virus might cause schizophrenia.

The viral hypothesis of schizophrenia has struck many scientists as a reasonable way of explaining several epidemiologic and clinical observations. Foremost among these is the finding that the births of individuals with schizophrenia are more likely to occur during the late winter and spring months than during other times of the year. Children born during these months are at increased risk for exposure to viruses while they are in the womb. Researchers reasoned that the effects of a virus at such an early age might alter the development of the brain in an abnormal direction. This 'season of birth effect' motivated the idea that a virus, toxic to the human brain, might be involved in the aetiology of some cases of schizophrenia. Interestingly, some studies found that the season of birth effect was strongest among patients without a family history of schizophrenia. Thus, it may be that viral cases of schizophrenia do not have a genetic origin, or that genetic factors are of lesser importance in such cases.

Although the season of birth effect is the most compelling evidence in favour of a viral cause of schizophrenia, other facts are also consistent with this theory. First, if a virus attacking the developing brain of a fetus causes schizophrenia, we would expect to observe other evidence of such effects. Two such effects have been seen in schizophrenia. First, individuals with schizophrenia have higher rates of physical anomalies. These are unusual characteristics in the shape of body parts. For example, facial deformities would be considered physical anomalies. Since physical anomalies can be caused by viruses that attack the fetus, the high rate of anomalies among individuals with schizophrenia supports the viral hypothesis. Second, some individuals with schizophrenia have unusual fingerprints. Although both physical anomalies and unusual fingerprints could be caused by PDCs or genetic abnormalities, their presence in schizophrenia could be the calling card from a viral attack on the brain.

The viral theory of schizophrenia has also been tested in studies of persons born during influenza epidemics. Since the influenza virus can create defects in the brain, fetuses exposed to the virus should have a higher risk for schizophrenia. One study examined adults in Finland who had been fetuses during a 1957 epidemic of influenza. Those adults who had been exposed to the epidemic during months 4, 5, or 6 of their mothers' pregnancy were at increased risk for subsequently being diagnosed with schizophrenia. This strongly suggests that the influenza virus contributed to schizophrenia risk in some people. However, a Scottish study failed to consistently find an increased risk for schizophrenia associated with influenza epidemics in 1918, 1919, or 1957, and only limited evidence of an association between viral epidemics and schizophrenia was found in an American study. Although the Finnish results were supported in a Danish sample, more research is needed to definitively conclude that viral infection during fetal development is a cause of schizophrenia.

Studies of 'familial' and 'sporadic' schizophrenia

As we have alluded to above, some studies of biological environmental factors have found that cases of 'sporadic' schizophrenia may exist. The word **sporadic** refers to cases that do not have a familial origin. Hence, the illness occurs only rarely (sporadically) within a given family. In contrast, **familial** schizophrenia refers to cases of the illness that co-occur with other cases in the same family. We and others use the word 'familial' instead of 'genetic' because illness may cluster in families for non-genetic reasons. Nevertheless, we believe that most cases of familial schizophrenia are indeed of a genetic origin, or have some genetic contribution.

The familial/sporadic point of view is an alternative to the diathesis-stress theory discussed above. The basic idea here is that schizophrenia may be caused by either genetic or environmental factors. For example, one type of schizophrenia might be due to a single gene or (more likely) a group of risk genes, but another could be caused by a virus. This may explain why it has been so difficult for researchers to definitively find a single cause for the disease. At our current stage of knowledge there is no infallible method for distinguishing between genetic and non-genetic forms of the illness. However, we can classify patients as either familial or sporadic. Patients having one or more relatives with schizophrenia are called familial. Those with no ill relatives are identified as sporadic. Of course, the categories familial and sporadic are not perfect indicators of the genetic and non-genetic categories, as they are based on self-report and limited knowledge of the familial pattern of illness. However, from any differences between familial and sporadic cases we may reasonably infer sources of genetic and environmental risk.

Familial and sporadic individuals with schizophrenia do not differ in age, sex, or clinical aspects of the illness, such as symptoms, age at onset, and need for hospitalization. In contrast, there are differences in measures of brain functioning. Most notably, difficulties sustaining attention are more common among familial schizophrenic patients. These patients find it difficult to perform tasks that require them to focus on an object for long periods of time. In other words, they are distractible; their attention is easily diverted to other aspects of the world around them. Patients with sporadic schizophrenia are more likely to have structural brain abnormalities when they are examined with methods like **computerized axial tomography (CAT) scans** or **magnetic resonance imaging (MRI)** that take pictures of brain structures. The abnormalities we refer to here indicate that the brains of sporadic patients show evidence of atrophy or loss of brain cells. Also, PDCs and winter births tend to be more common among sporadic cases of schizophrenia compared with familial cases. We cannot draw strong conclusions from these studies because, although most support these findings, some do not. Nevertheless, the available results fit well with the idea that adverse environmental events can impact neurodevelopment which leads to a non-genetic form of schizophrenia.

Another approach for identifying patients with possible genetic and environmental forms of an illness requires the comparison of concordant and discordant monozygotic (MZ) twins. If twins are MZ, then their genes are identical. Thus, if a trait is completely determined by genetic factors, both twins should express it. Given these facts, MZ twin pairs that are concordant for schizophrenia are more likely to have a genetic form of schizophrenia. In contrast, MZ pairs discordant for the illness might have an environmental form of schizophrenia. Researchers at the Maudsley Hospital in London, England, examined 21 MZ pairs: nine were concordant for schizophrenia, and 12 were discordant. There were no differences in measures of structural brain abnormalities between the affected members of discordant and concordant pairs. However, those without a family history of schizophrenia had more brain atrophy. These researchers also found more pregnancy and delivery complications among the individuals with schizophrenia who belonged to the discordant MZ pairs.

If twins are discordant because of an environmental cause of schizophrenia, then only the relatives of *concordant* pairs should be at increased risk for the illness. While some studies find this result, others do not. These studies indicate that some of the twins in discordant pairs have a genetic illness. How large the sporadic subset might be is not known.

In summary, studies of familial and sporadic individuals with schizophrenia have produced mixed results. Some are consistent with the idea that there are non-genetic forms of schizophrenia. It seems likely that PDCs are responsible for some of these apparently non-genetic cases. Another possibility is advanced paternal age, which increases the risk for schizophrenia among the offspring. The mechanism for this relationship may be the breakdown of DNA repair mechanisms with age, allowing more mutations to accrue in sperm made later in life and thus those mutations are passed on to offspring. In this scenario, the father (and the remainder of the family) may have no personal history of schizophrenia, but genes still play a role in the schizophrenia that develops in the child. The role of viruses or other environmental factors is not proven or settled. These studies cannot rule out the diathesis–stress model of schizophrenia discussed earlier. In fact, some of these studies are more consistent with this theory than they are with the proposition that some non-genetic forms exist. More research is needed to choose between these two ideas or to determine which cases of schizophrenia are due to each type of cause.

Studies of the prodromal period of high risk for schizophrenia

Another set of studies has focused on young adults deemed to be at ultra-high risk for psychosis, including schizophrenia. This designation includes symptoms of the schizophrenia prodrome and is thought to signal the imminent descent of functioning toward the levels required for a schizophrenia diagnosis. These 44 studies show that people at ultra-high risk for psychosis (but not yet with schizophrenia) were more likely to have had PDCs, drug and alcohol use, physical inactivity, childhood trauma, emotional abuse, or physical neglect, and high perceived stress. These ultra-high risk studies are valuable for evaluating if these well-known associations with schizophrenia come before schizophrenia and possibly play a role in its emergence, or are simply effects of becoming ill. The existing data suggest that such environmental risk factors may, indeed, pose risks for the development of schizophrenia, but it is possible that these are outcomes (like schizophrenia itself) of an underlying genetic or biological risk state.

Summary

Several environmental factors are reliably associated with schizophrenia. It is often hard to tell if these associated environmental factors come before the disorder and contribute to its development, or are merely events that go hand in hand with the emergence of schizophrenia symptoms. Studies of children who grow up to develop schizophrenia, and studies of young adults at ultra-high risk for schizophrenia, give us the best chance to determine if these environmental factors are causal or just correlations. These studies do not largely provide support for psychosocial factors—such as parenting styles or socioeconomic conditions—leading to schizophrenia. In contrast, several biological environmental factors do have support as causal factors. Substance abuse, childhood trauma, PDCs, and even paternal age are all verified environmental risk factors for schizophrenia. Advancing paternal age is thought to allow more genetic mutations to accumulate in sperm and pass on to offspring, heightening their risk. These biological environmental factors increase the risk for schizophrenia by about 30–100% beyond the baseline risk (so perhaps moving an individual's risk from the population rate of 1% to approximately 1.3–2%), so are relatively small risk factors. It is unlikely that any of these factors would be sufficient to cause schizophrenia on its own in most cases; instead, such environmental factors probably need to interact with each other and with risk genes to cause someone to develop the disorder.

8

Is schizophrenia a brain disorder?

> ## ➲ Key points
>
> ◆ Brain-imaging studies have found brain atrophy in 20–50% of individuals with schizophrenia.
>
> ◆ Individuals with schizophrenia have less metabolic activity in some parts of the brain, suggesting that the brain of individuals with schizophrenia cannot react to stimuli as effectively as a normal brain.
>
> ◆ Blood flow to the frontal cortex is lower in individuals with schizophrenia, and these individuals also perform poorly on tests of attention, motor function, and abstraction (all functions of the frontal cortex).
>
> ◆ Individuals with schizophrenia have more left-brain dysfunction (as measured by language and writing tasks) than right-brain dysfunction (as measured by spatial tasks).
>
> ◆ The dopamine theory states that overactivity of a brain chemical called dopamine may cause schizophrenia. While this theory is too simple, many signs suggest that having too much dopamine is probably one of the brain defects leading to schizophrenia.

In the language of psychiatry, disorders that change the functioning of psychological processes or emotion are called either 'symptomatic' or 'idiopathic'. **Symptomatic** disorders are those for which there is a known physical cause. For example, temporal lobe epilepsy, strokes, and brain tumours can change mental functioning and emotional expression. In these cases, the physical cause can be found by using electroencephalograms (which measure the electrical activity of the brain), X-rays, or similar, but more sophisticated, methods of assessment. In contrast, we say a disorder is **idiopathic** if it has no *known* physical cause. We emphasize the word 'known' because most scientists expect that physical causes of schizophrenia will some day be found when we can look more closely at the molecular level. The term 'idiopathic' originally reflected the belief that these disorders were due to psychological and social events that had no physical effects on the brain.

When the first edition of this book was published, psychiatry was undergoing a revolution in its approach to mental illness, especially schizophrenia. Many scientists and clinicians were starting to question the idea that schizophrenia was rooted in psychological and family conflict. Instead, they thought that the massive alterations in thought and emotion in people with schizophrenia were due to a disease of the brain.

This chapter reviews evidence showing that biological processes are altered in the brains of individuals with schizophrenia. During the past century, scientists have created many methods for studying the brain. As each of these new neuroimaging technologies emerged, they were swiftly applied to the study of schizophrenia. As we shall see, most of these measurements led to the same conclusion: that the structure and function of the brains of some individuals with schizophrenia were not normal. We are, however, still uncertain about many of the details of the **aetiology** and **pathophysiology** of the disorder. Aetiology refers to the causes of brain dysfunction (e.g., defective genes, environmental risk factors); pathophysiology denotes the specific modifications of the brain that lead to illness (e.g., brain atrophy, too much dopamine). For example, a variant of a gene that influences the activity of brain cells might be part of the aetiology of schizophrenia, while the corresponding pathophysiology might be atrophy of the brain as measured by a brain scan.

Structural brain abnormalities

We use the phrase 'structural brain abnormalities' to refer to any unusual changes in the form or configuration of the brain observed in individuals with schizophrenia but not in healthy people. The most direct way to see such changes is to look at the brain, after death, using methods from neuropathology. Many such studies have been done thanks to the generosity of individuals who agreed to donate their brain to research following their deaths. We can draw two major conclusions from the results of these neuropathological studies of schizophrenia. First, abnormalities of the brain are common in individuals with schizophrenia. Second, researchers have not found a single abnormality that is found in all or even most brains from individuals with schizophrenia. This is a curious result, which we will see mirrored by other methods of studying the schizophrenic brain. Whereas most well-defined brain diseases leave a distinct pathophysiological 'signature' on the brain, this is not the case for schizophrenia. This complexity does, however, mirror what we know of the genetics of schizophrenia, where we learned that no single gene is either necessary or sufficient to cause the disorder.

Neuropathology studies of *post-mortem* brain are difficult to do because we must wait for the patient's death before studying the brain. Fortunately, several methods allow us to study the structure of the brain in living patients. These methods are called 'imaging' techniques because they provide us with an image of the living brain. They are similar to the simple X-ray procedure that most of us have experienced in our doctor's office. Like the X-ray, these imaging methods create a picture of the brain that can be used to find abnormalities.

Structural abnormalities have been found in a large number of brain regions in people with schizophrenia, from *post-mortem* tissue analysis and structural brain imaging techniques such as computer-assisted tomography (CAT), magnetic resonance imaging (MRI), and diffusion tensor imaging (DTI). A growing consensus is building for those brain structures that have been most often seen as disrupted in schizophrenia. Larger volume of the lateral ventricles is often observed, as well as decreases in the size of the dorsolateral and medial prefrontal cortices (the outer parts of the front of the brain), cingulate and paracingulate cortices (middle parts of the brain), hippocampus, amygdala, parahippocampal and superior temporal gyri (side of the brain), septum pellucidum, and thalamus (deep parts of the brain). More precisely, positive symptoms of schizophrenia have been found to associate with thinning of the cortex in the superior temporal gyrus, while negative symptoms are correlated with thinning of the prefrontal cortex. These abnormalities of brain structure may be core features of the disorder or, at the very least, are among the most common and most severe structural brain abnormalities among schizophrenic patients.

In 1927, a method known as 'pneumoencephalography' found that 18 of 19 individuals with schizophrenia had enlarged ventricles. Ventricles are spaces within the brain containing fluid, but not solid brain substance. Ventricles enlarge when the brain substance that surrounds them loses brain cells. We refer to this loss of brain cells as 'atrophy'. Thus, patients with larger ventricles have fewer brain cells. This early finding was confirmed in subsequent pneumoencephalographic studies. Unfortunately, these pioneering findings were largely ignored since psychological theories of schizophrenia were in vogue.

Psychiatry rediscovered brain atrophy in schizophrenia in 1976 when Drs Eva Johnstone and Timothy Crow and colleagues of the British Medical Research Council Clinical Research Centre reported larger ventricles in patients with schizophrenia who were studied with the imaging method known as CAT. The CAT scanner takes pictures of the living brain in small 'slices'. This allowed researchers to see the inner portions of the brain more accurately than had been previously possible. In the 1980s the method of MRI was also applied to schizophrenia. MRI scans provide a three-dimensional image of the living brain in a manner that allows us to see more of the details of brain structure than had been possible with the CAT scan. Many CAT scan and MRI scan studies of schizophrenia confirmed that many individuals with schizophrenia have larger ventricles than normal. In fact, a 2010 review of structural neuroimaging studies done over time has also shown that the enlargement of ventricles in schizophrenia grows over the course of many years, suggesting that the disorder may not just emerge as a developmental process, but may involve brain cell death too. In addition to ventricular enlargement, several MRI studies report reduced size of specific regions of the brain in schizophrenia. For example, a 2005 review of all structural MRI studies of schizophrenia found that as many as 50 discrete brain regions showed some volume change (usually decrease in size) in individuals with schizophrenia relative to healthy comparison subjects. The brain regions found most consistently to be abnormally structured in schizophrenia included the left superior temporal gyrus and the left medial temporal lobe. Later, a recent very large meta-analysis of deep structures of the brain also found reliable decreases in the size of the hippocampus, amygdala, thalamus, and the nucleus accumbens, while confirming larger lateral ventricle size in individuals with schizophrenia.

More work is needed to pinpoint all regions of tissue loss in the brain and to determine the significance of large ventricles for people with schizophrenia, and other challenges remain. Although, as a group, individuals with schizophrenia have larger ventricles than normal, many individuals with schizophrenia have normal ventricles. Depending on the group of patients studied, only 20–50% of individuals with schizophrenia will have enlarged ventricles. However, when it does occur, the ventricular enlargement associated with schizophrenia is present at and even before the onset of the illness. Thus, it is not a side effect of repeated hospitalization, drug treatment, or other factors associated with schizophrenia.

Patients with enlarged ventricles differ from other patients in several ways. They tend to have more negative symptoms such as flatness of emotion and social withdrawal. They are also more likely to have trouble thinking, as measured by neuropsychological tests. In many ways, their illness appears to be more severe. They usually cannot live alone but require either permanent hospitalization or the structure of a halfway house or foster home. When they are hospitalized, they require relatively long hospital stays and do not respond well to most treatment programmes. Also, as noted in a previous chapter, ventricular enlargement is more common among individuals with schizophrenia without a family history of schizophrenia. These results initially suggested that enlarged ventricles might identify a subtype of schizophrenia. However, researchers have not yet been able to isolate a consistent subtype with this feature. Moreover, ventricular enlargement is not limited to schizophrenia. It has also been reported in other psychiatric disorders including bipolar disorder, schizoaffective disorder, and obsessive-compulsive disorder.

The integrity of brain structure in schizoaffective disorder has not received much research attention independent from schizophrenia; rather, patients with schizoaffective disorder are usually examined jointly with individuals with schizophrenia, reflecting the similarity of the two on the continuum of clinical features and aetiology. Yet, the few studies that have looked at the state of the brain in schizoaffective disorder have provided largely supportive evidence for common morphology in the two disorders. For example, ventricular enlargement (which is characteristic of schizophrenia) has been observed in most studies of schizoaffective disorder. Schizoaffective disorder is also marked by size deficits in frontal and temporal lobes of the cortex, the striatum, the fusiform gyrus, the cuneus and precuneus, and the lingual and limbic regions. Much more work is needed in this area.

Schizotypal personality disorder has been thought of as a related and less severe version of schizophrenia. In support of that, many (but not all) of the structural abnormalities present in schizophrenia are also apparent in schizotypal personality disorder. For example, individuals with schizotypal personality disorder show brain abnormalities in the medial temporal lobe, superior and parahippocampal gyri, lateral ventricles, thalamus, and septum pellucidum that are similar to those seen in persons with schizophrenia. Of note, a 2013 meta-analysis of MRI studies of the two disorders found that, in contrast to the prefrontal cortex shrinkage seen in schizophrenia, this region was larger in individuals with schizotypal personality disorder. It is unclear if this enlargement is some form of protective or compensatory mechanism.

Structural brain imaging and post-mortem tissue analysis is rare for schizoid or paranoid personality disorders, but one MRI study of schizoid personality disorder found an increase in the size of the superior part of the corona radiate in those affected with the disorder. The psychosis-risk state (which, after Paul Meehl, we reconceptualized as '**schizotaxia**') has received some attention, and findings of structural abnormalities in the non-psychotic relatives of individuals with schizophrenia are now becoming widely recognized too. Compared with unaffected individuals, this subgroup of relatives has brain size decreases in the amygdala-hippocampal region, thalamus, and cerebellum, and significantly increased volumes in the pallidum. Schizotaxic relatives of individuals with schizophrenia may also show lower volumes in other medial limbic and paralimbic structures, including the anterior cingulate and paracingulate cortex, insula, and parahippocampal gyrus.

While structural MRI can help measure the size of brain regions, DTI measures a different aspect of brain structure. DTI helps scientists see how intact or disrupted the connections are between brain regions. DTI is a relatively new technology that measures the degree to which the brain's 'white matter' or nerve fibres (as opposed to 'grey matter' or cells) is intact. In a typical brain, the connections between brain regions are orderly, to allow efficient cross-talk. In schizophrenia, however, these nerve fibres are very widely disrupted throughout the brain. A comprehensive review of DTI studies of schizophrenia showed that a large majority of them had found reduced 'anisotropy' in affected individuals compared to unaffected control subjects. A reduction in anisotropy is taken to indicate that the nerve fibres in a particular tract are not properly aligned, and may reflect aberrations in axonal branching or projection which could lead to inefficient transmission of nerve impulses between brain regions. Despite the high degree of uniformity found at the level of global anisotropy reductions in schizophrenia, until recently there had been very little agreement between studies about the particular tracts in the brain where deficits are most pronounced or most reliably detected. A relatively new meta-analysis of 53 studies found disruptions of long projection fibres, corpus callosal and commissural fibres (which allow communication between the different sides of the brain), part of motor descending fibres, and fronto-temporal-limbic pathways. Collectively, MRI and DTI studies paint a picture of schizophrenia that involves shrinkage of numerous brain regions, and disordered connectivity between brain regions. These brain changes, or any portion of these, occurring in an individual with schizophrenia would be expected to have some negative impact on brain processes, which we review next.

Abnormalities of brain functioning

Whereas studies of brain *structure* look at the physical form, configuration, and connections of the brain, studies of brain *function* examine whether the brain is working correctly, regardless of its overall structure. A simple analogy helps to clarify the difference between brain structure and function. Consider an automobile engine that will not start. If a part, say the battery, is missing we conclude that the structure of the engine is abnormal. In contrast, if the battery is weak and the spark plugs are dirty, we conclude that despite its normal structure, the engine has two specific defects in functioning.

The ability to study brain functioning in living people is perhaps one of the great contributions of neuroscience. To study the activity of the living brain, without harming the subject, was a monumental challenge. Fortunately, breakthroughs in medical technology have now made this possible. In fact, several methods of observing brain functioning were invented. Each of these suggests that individuals with schizophrenia have abnormalities of brain function.

In studies of regional cerebral blood flow (RCBF), scientists measure the amount of blood that is flowing to specific regions of the brain. Since the brain requires an ongoing supply of blood to work well, less blood flow indicates potential problems with brain functioning. Total brain blood flow is reduced in schizophrenia, and regional blood flow results suggest a particular reduction in blood flow to the frontal cortex. The frontal cortex is the large portion of the brain at its front. It controls many aspects of human thought and emotion. In many ways, it is the brain's supervisor because it coordinates and integrates the activities of other brain centres.

Positron emission tomography (PET) uses radioactive substances to measure the metabolism of the sugar glucose by specific parts of the brain. Since brain cells use glucose to function, less glucose use may indicate decreases in brain functioning. PET studies confirmed the findings of RCBF studies by showing a relative reduction in metabolic activity in the frontal cortex of individuals with schizophrenia. These reductions were most notable when the patient performed a mental task during the procedure. This suggests that the brain, in schizophrenia, cannot react to the world around it as quickly or as efficiently as a healthy brain. A meta-analysis of 155 studies on this topic found that this '**hypofrontality**' may be seen in approximately half of individuals with schizophrenia.

Some investigators think that the left side of the brain is particularly dysfunctional in individuals with schizophrenia. Originally this idea came from observations of one particular type of epilepsy (temporal epilepsy) in which abnormal brain waves arise from the temporal lobes at the sides of the brain. The word 'lobe' means 'region of the brain.' Sufferers from this form of epilepsy sometimes have symptoms that can't be distinguished from those of true schizophrenia. It seems that the temporal lobes may be involved in the production of certain schizophrenia symptoms such as delusions, hallucinations, or disorganized thoughts. Furthermore, temporal lobe epilepsy in primarily the left side of the brain tends to show more schizophrenia features, such as disorganized thoughts, whereas temporal epilepsy in the right side of the brain more often shows symptoms of mood disorder. This led to an intriguing idea: perhaps the left side of the brain was impaired in schizophrenia.

In support of this idea were reports that a fairly high proportion of individuals with schizophrenia are left-handed. This finding is relevant as most people are right-handed because the left side of their brain is dominant to the right side. Since the left brain controls the right hand (and the right brain controls the left hand), left-handedness may indicate that the left side of the brain is not functioning properly and therefore has lost its dominance over the right brain. This idea has received much attention because the left side of the brain controls language and thought, and these are impaired in schizophrenia. Visual or spatial abilities (a function of the right brain) are not as often or severely impaired in the disorder.

Overall, RCBF and PET studies lend some support to the idea that individuals with schizophrenia have a dysfunctional left brain and that they fail to shift mental processing to the right brain when needed. For example, one study found that the relative amount of blood flow to the left and right brains differentiated patients with schizophrenia from people without psychiatric problems. For a verbal task (controlled by the left brain), the patients showed no flow asymmetries, but the healthy subjects showed an increase in left brain flow. For a spatial task (controlled by the right brain) the patients showed greater left brain increases than right brain increases; the healthy subjects showed a larger right brain increase on the same task.

Another approach to brain imaging has been to look at the electrical activity of the brain. Since nerve cells in the brain communicate with electrical–chemical impulses, methods that measure the pattern of electrical activity can help understand brain functioning. The electroencephalogram (EEG) has a long history of use in schizophrenia studies. In the popular press, the EEG is often reported as the study of 'brain waves' because it records the electrical activity of the brain in a series of wavy signal lines. Twenty to 40% of individuals with schizophrenia have EEG recordings that are abnormal. These abnormalities are not related to the clinical features of the patients, their duration of illness, or the severity of their illness. The EEG abnormalities are usually observed on both the left and right sides of the brain. These deviant EEG patterns are not only seen in schizophrenia; we also see them in other psychiatric and neurological patients. However, the type of abnormality seen among individuals with schizophrenia differs from the epileptiform activity seen in patients with epilepsy.

Most recent functional neuroimaging studies that produce reliable facts about the brain in schizophrenia involve functional MRI (fMRI). fMRI couples the techniques of MRI described above, in our review of structural brain abnormalities, and RCBF to spatially localize abnormal brain energy use patterns in discrete brain regions during the performance of a particular task. Usually, the task is picked or designed to draw largely on one or a few regions of the brain. This technique has even been used recently in the resting state to identify abnormalities in the so-called 'default network' in schizophrenia, which is a large group of brain structures that are active when an individual is not actively attending to or interacting with the outside world. This suggests that functional neurobiological problems in schizophrenia are present not only when the brain is taxed, but also when it is at rest. Consistent with other imaging modalities, the most routinely observed fMRI abnormalities in schizophrenia include a decrease in frontal lobe activity ('hypofrontality') during the performance of demanding cognitive tasks. More recently, some data have emerged to suggest that overall activity in the frontal lobes is not reduced but simply more dispersed in individuals with schizophrenia, suggesting less efficient processing and the notion that the brain must work harder in individuals with schizophrenia to attain normal levels of performance.

Collectively, functional studies of schizophrenia find abnormal patterns of brain activation that are confined to those regions in which structural abnormalities have also been noted. The same may be true for the spectrum conditions as well, although, some anomalies in structure and function do not overlap in schizophrenia. It has been somewhat difficult to integrate all of the reports of functional brain abnormalities in schizophrenia due to methodological considerations. Most importantly, patterns of brain activation are influenced by the demands placed on the individuals during the imaging process. Thus, functional brain images taken from people with schizophrenia performing a wide variety of tasks in different studies (e.g., a working memory task, an auditory vigilance task, and a verbal comprehension test) are not readily combinable. Furthermore, large, reliable studies specifically seeking similar deficits on consistently impaired processes in schizophrenia (e.g., motor task performance, verbal fluency, auditory attention, working memory) in patients with schizoaffective disorder or schizoid or paranoid personality disorders have yet to emerge. Although functional brain imaging is a powerful tool, it has yet to influence our understanding of most schizophrenia-spectrum disorders and their treatment, although there is little doubt that it will work soon.

The exception to this generalization is schizotypal personality disorder, for which a small but important body of work exists. These reports of functional abnormalities in schizotypal personality disorder are so important because the picture that emerges seems to further justify the personality disorder's position along the schizophrenia spectrum. For example, some work finds that abnormalities in frontal activation in schizotypal personality disorder mimic those of schizophrenia, but that alternative brain regions are recruited by schizotypal personality-disordered individuals to help accomplish tasks requiring frontal lobe activation.

Genetic heterogeneity and brain dysfunction in schizophrenia

The lack of necessary or sufficient environmental or genetic causes for schizophrenia has been taken as evidence for genetic heterogeneity in the causation of the disorder. This conclusion suggests that several genetic forms of schizophrenia may exist, along with some non-genetic forms as well. A theoretical distinction has been made between people with schizophrenia having a family history of the disorder (familial cases) and those with no such family history (sporadic cases). Furthermore, some studies find that this division is valid and useful for identifying specific deficits that may be heritable. For example, measures of attention, particularly sustained attention or vigilance as measured by the continuous performance test (CPT), are impaired more often in familial cases of schizophrenia than in sporadic cases. Furthermore, it is quite interesting to note that poor attentional performance is consistently observed in the relatives of individuals with schizophrenia. However, differences in attention between familial and sporadic cases of schizophrenia are not always found, and people with familial schizophrenia outperform sporadic people with schizophrenia on a different measure of attention, the digit span task.

Evidence from electrophysiologic studies of the brains of people with schizophrenia suggests that these differences in attention between familial and sporadic cases may have a neurobiological basis. For example, familial cases are more likely to have abnormal brain waves in response to sounds of images. Also, some relatives of individuals with schizophrenia demonstrate the same evoked-potential abnormalities. Thus, the relatives of individuals with schizophrenia show abnormalities in tests of sustained attention and in evoked-potential recordings, deficits that were also found more often in familial cases of schizophrenia than in non-familial cases. In contrast, irregular EEGs are detected more frequently in sporadic cases than in familial cases.

The weight of evidence supports the notion that sporadic cases of schizophrenia exhibit more structural brain abnormalities than familial cases. This difference substantiated earlier work that found no difference in the ventricular size between concordant and discordant MZ twin-pairs, but significantly larger ventricles in patients with no family history of the illness. Subsequently, the ventricular–brain ratio was found to be 21% greater in subjects with no family history of schizophrenia than in subjects with a positive family history of the disorder. Thus, the body of work indicates that there is an increase in ventricular volume in at least some non-familial individuals with schizophrenia.

The evidence for increased brain abnormalities in non-familial cases of schizophrenia suggests a major role for environmental factors in their aetiology. This hypothesis is further supported by findings from twin studies in which the affected members of discordant MZ twin-pairs were found to have greater neurodiagnostic abnormalities than their unaffected co-twins. Specifically, the affected siblings had greater neuropsychological dysfunction, larger cerebral ventricles, more abnormalities in brain MRIs, and greater 'hypofrontality'. Because MZ twins are genetically identical, such differences between the members of these twin-pairs must be due to environmental factors.

Dr Tyrone Cannon first proposed that obstetric complications (OCs) might combine with the genetic predisposition to schizophrenia to produce these structural brain abnormalities. Within a high-risk sample, there were clear increases in the ratios of cortex and ventricular cerebrospinal fluid to whole brain as the level of genetic liability to schizophrenia increased. Furthermore, the effect of OCs on ventricular size increased as the level of genetic risk for schizophrenia increased, such that OCs had little effect on this measure in subjects with two normal parents, a larger effect in those with one affected parent, and the largest impact on those individuals with two affected parents.

A full understanding of the aetiology and pathophysiology of schizophrenia is obscured by the heterogeneity of the disorder. However, this obstacle may be overcome if more intensive research efforts are directed at this issue. Currently, attempts are being made to isolate homogeneous subgroups of individuals with schizophrenia based on clinical features, neurobiological measures, and even based on genetic subgroups. Ultimately this work may help our understanding of the course and outcome of schizophrenia, as well as the role of psychosocial factors in these processes. Changes in diagnostic systems coming from this work should also improve the ability of clinicians to choose the most effective treatment regimens for different subgroups of individuals with schizophrenia. Until these goals have been realized, the most effective treatment of schizophrenia spectrum disorders must continue to be derived from an extensive knowledge of the individual patient, clinical skill, and compassion.

Neuropsychological measures of brain functioning

The physiological measures of brain functioning discussed above provide clear evidence that the brain does not function entirely correctly in schizophrenia. However, because they measure physical aspects of the brain, they tell us little about how brain abnormalities in schizophrenia affect the patient's behaviour. The study of how brain abnormalities affect behaviour is a subspecialty of psychology known as 'neuropsychology'. In a neuropsychological study of schizophrenia, the neuropsychologist asks the patient to perform many tasks. These tasks are designed to measure specific aspects of brain functioning. For example, to test verbal memory, the neuropsychologist may read a story and then ask the patient questions to see if key points are remembered. To test visual memory, we show the patient designs and see if they can be recalled.

Most of us are familiar with the concept of intelligence. To a neuropsychologist, intelligence summarizes a person's overall level of brain functioning. In lay terms, it tells us how smart a person is when asked to do mental tasks. Individuals with schizophrenia perform more poorly than healthy subjects on standardized intelligence tests. *On average,* the intelligence quotients (IQs) of individuals with schizophrenia are five to ten points lower than normal. We emphasize 'on average' because many patients with schizophrenia have normal IQs or even very high IQs (think John Nash, from *A Beautiful Mind*) and some healthy people have IQs lower than some affected individuals. Nevertheless, the lower average IQ scores of individuals with schizophrenia suggest that the abnormalities of brain structure and function discussed above lead to decreased abilities to perform mental tasks. The goal of neuropsychological studies has been to separate the abilities that are impaired in individuals with schizophrenia from those that are not.

Attention is a common word with many meanings to the layperson. The neuropsychologist breaks down the everyday idea of attention into several categories. **Immediate attention** is the ability to focus on a task for a short period. **Sustained attention** assesses the ability to focus on a task for a long period. We also speak of **selective attention**, the ability to focus on one thing (e.g., a conversation) while ignoring another (e.g., background music).

Individuals with schizophrenia show problems in each of these areas of attention. In general, their ability to pay attention worsens as the task becomes more difficult.

Motor abilities refer to the coordination of thinking and muscles to accomplish a task. One aspect of motor functioning is speed. How quickly can a task be done? In most studies, individuals with schizophrenia are consistently slower than normal. It is difficult for the neuropsychologist to know if this slowness is due to problems with attention or other abilities. Whatever the cause of this slow response speed, it makes it difficult for individuals with schizophrenia to work as efficiently as a healthy person. Thus, it is one of the many reasons they find it difficult to maintain steady employment.

Deficits in **abstraction** and **concept formation** have long been seen among individuals with schizophrenia. Both of these are necessary components of effective, higher level thinking. *Abstraction* is the ability to move from the specific, observable aspects of life to general principles. The most straightforward example is concept formation whereby we group items. This may be as simple as knowing that mice, cats, and dogs are all animals; but concept formation can be very complex, as in learning the boundaries of ethical behaviour. More importantly, these functions are closely related to the planning and organizational skills we need in everyday life. It is not surprising that many people with schizophrenia do poorly on these tasks since clinical observations show them to be deficient in many of these skills. Notably, their poor performance on these tasks is related to reduced activity of the frontal cortex measured in blood-flow studies of the brain. Thus, the neuropsychological studies are consistent with the imaging studies discussed above.

Our clinical descriptions of schizophrenia noted that thought disorder is a common symptom. Thus, it is not surprising that these patients also have problems with neuropsychological measures of **verbal ability** and **language**. Yet these problems are different from the speech and language problems that neurologists describe in many neurology patients. For example, individuals with schizophrenia usually have mild language problems in which simple language functions like naming objects and understanding speech are not affected. These simple functions are often disturbed in people with neurological conditions. In contrast, individuals with schizophrenia usually have problems with complex language tasks.

As we all know from everyday experience, **learning and memory** are essential mental activities, which we use on a regular basis. Research consistently finds that individuals with schizophrenia have difficulties with learning and memory. They have learning and memory problems for both verbal information (words, sentences, and stories) and visual information (pictures). In both these areas, the memory deficits are seen if affected individuals are asked to remember items over short or long periods of time.

Individuals with schizophrenia tend to do reasonably well on simple **visual–spatial** tasks. These tasks require the subject to observe a problem and find its solution based on the spatial relationships of items that are seen. For example, organizing a group of blocks to match a design is a visual–spatial task. Relative to other neuropsychological skills, visual–spatial functioning appears to be less impaired in schizophrenia. This finding may be related to the issue of **brain asymmetry**. This is a complicated issue since it involves knowledge of how the normal human brain is organized. A simplified, yet essentially correct, description is as follows. The brain is composed of two halves, left and right, which look very similar to one another. After cutting an orange in half, the two halves look like one another. We say the orange is symmetrical. The human brain, with some exceptions, is physically symmetrical. However, it is functionally asymmetrical. By this, we mean that the left and right brains control different mental tasks. Most notably, the left brain is responsible for processing language. It thinks in a logical, sequential manner. In contrast, the right brain processes non-linguistic material. We use it for visual–spatial and other tasks that require us to think 'without language'. For example, if we ask you to copy a design, you are likely to make the copy without talking to yourself about the specific features of the design you are copying. When a mental function is performed by one half of the brain, we say that the function is 'lateralized' or exhibits 'brain laterality'.

Neurotransmitter dysfunction

The studies we have discussed so far show that the brains of individuals with schizophrenia do not function correctly. They do not, however, tell us the causes of this dysfunction. For example, we do not believe that decreased blood flow, abnormal glucose use, or neuropsychological phenomena cause schizophrenia. Instead, they are best thought of as markers of brain function that are affected by the disease process that causes schizophrenia. Ideally, we would know what causes these brain abnormalities since that might lead us to the ultimate cause of schizophrenia.

Many scientists have proposed that the underlying cause of schizophrenia can be found within the neurotransmitter systems of the brain. To make this clear, we must provide a brief overview of how these systems work. The brain is composed of thousands of brain cells called neurons. These neurons collect information from the five senses and relay it to other neurons in the brain for mental processing. These neurons, in turn, may relay the information to one or more areas of the brain for additional mental processing. To relay information, a neuron must send a chemical message to another neuron.

Neurons are separated by a small gap called the 'synapse'. To send a message to the second neuron, the first one must release a chemical called a neurotransmitter. This neurotransmitter travels across the synapse and eventually lands on little platforms, called receptors, which are attached to the second neuron.

When enough of these platforms are occupied, an electrical signal is created in the second neuron that corresponds to the message being sent. When the size of this electrical signal exceeds a threshold, an electrical impulse is sent across the second neuron. In this manner, the neurons in the brain talk to one another and control all the functions of our mind and body (Figure 8.1).

The chemical communication of the synapse is a remarkable system that usually works very efficiently. However, there are several ways in which a disease can interfere with this process. For example, the first neuron may not produce enough chemical, it may produce too much chemical, or it may produce the wrong chemical. A problem could also occur with the second neuron. It may not have enough receptors, or it may have too many. Also, if the shape of the receptor is wrong, then the chemical released by the first neuron might not be able to land. Thus, a common theme of the neurotransmitter theories of schizophrenia is that imbalances in the concentration of neurotransmitters or abnormal activities at the synapse cause the illness.

Although many functional imaging methods measure 'brain activation' by quantifying energy consumption, the functional abnormalities in the brains of

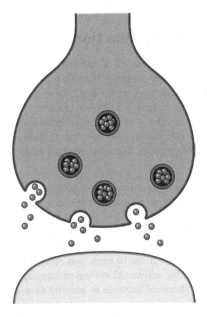

Figure 8.1 Neuron and Synapse.
Reproduced under the terms of the Creative Commons Attribution 3.0 Unported license (CC BY 3.0), https://creativecommons.org/licenses/by/3.0/ from Smart Servier Medical Art,https://smart.servier.com/

individuals with schizophrenia do not simply reflect a different pattern of blood flow or oxygenation, or glucose utilization (although these may be indicated). Rather, these differences are thought to be the observable consequence of altered neurotransmission. Thus, by proxy, functional brain imaging changes give some indication of underlying neurochemical and neurophysiological pathology.

For decades, the central dopamine systems were considered the prime neural substrates of schizophrenia symptoms, and with good reason; the evidence supporting dopaminergic problems in schizophrenia is vast. The 'dopamine hypothesis' of schizophrenia pathology was derived chiefly from observations that typical antipsychotic medications blocked dopamine D2 receptors, while indirect dopamine stimulators like amphetamine produced psychotic symptoms that look like those of schizophrenia. The initial and most basic form of the dopamine hypothesis asserted that schizophrenia results from dopaminergic hyperactivity, i.e. too much dopamine. Later reformulations focused on relationships between hyperactivity in mesolimbic dopamine neurons and dopaminergic hypoactivity in the prefrontal cortex (contributing to hypofrontality). Although a solely dopaminergic hypothesis of schizophrenia is likely to be too simplistic to explain the development of the disorder, there is much evidence for both cortical dopaminergic hypoactivity and subcortical dopaminergic hyperactivity in schizophrenia.

Neuroimaging techniques offer perhaps the best current methods for testing aspects of neurotransmission non-invasively. Methods such as positron emission tomography and single-photon emission computerized tomography are not capable of visualizing actual neurotransmission but can provide indirect measures of these by selectively measuring the receptor activity in specific neurotransmitter pathways. The application of such methods has shown that dopamine transporter occupancy is not altered in schizophrenia, even early in the disease process, or in patients experiencing their first psychotic episode. Dopamine D2 receptors, however, have been reliably found to be occupied to a greater extent in individuals with schizophrenia than in healthy subjects, and at least a subset of patients exhibits greater D2 receptor numbers. Serotonin 2A receptors do not appear to be reliably altered in the brain in schizophrenia, and a very recent meta-analysis 23 imaging studies also found no reliable evidence for the involvement of gamma-amino butyric acid A (GABA) receptors either.

The diversity of clinical symptoms in schizophrenia, the overwhelming evidence for a complex genetic aetiology, the multiple neurochemical actions of atypical antipsychotic medications such as clozapine, and the demonstration of numerous neurochemical and brain structure abnormalities all underlie the view that multiple biochemical deficits contribute to schizophrenia. Thus, aside from dopaminergic dysfunction, abnormalities in glutamate neurotransmission are becoming central to working hypotheses of the pathology of schizophrenia. Much of this attention is derived from the fact that glutamate is a ubiquitous excitatory neurotransmitter in the central nervous system, which allows it to interact with many other transmitter systems, including dopamine (thus, dopamine dysfunction is presumed to follow from glutamatergic dysfunction). N-methyl-d-aspartate (NMDA) and α-amino-3-hydroxy-5-methyl-4-isoxasolepropionate glutamate receptors in the nucleus accumbens modulate dopaminergic neurons in the nucleus accumbens and the frontal cortex, but the effect of glutamate differs at the two sites. The presence of presynaptic glutamate receptors on dopamine neurons in the frontal cortex results in facilitation of dopamine function, while dopamine reuptake is inhibited and release facilitated by glutamate in the nucleus accumbens. This means that agents that interfere with glutamate transmission would facilitate cortical dopaminergic hypoactivity and subcortical hyperactivity, which is consistent with the dopamine hypothesis of schizophrenia.

Further evidence for a role of glutamate in schizophrenia is derived from the fact that it is a critical neural substrate of cortical-level processing and cognition. Also, manipulations of glutamatergic function in schizophrenia reduce negative symptoms and improve cognition. In fact, glutamatergic antagonists, such as phencyclidine, bring on psychotic symptoms from non-schizophrenic individuals that resemble the illness, and they exacerbate symptoms in individuals with schizophrenia. Phencyclidine acts by binding to a site on the NMDA receptor that blocks the influx of calcium and other cations through the ion channel, which then blocks receptor function. The effects of NMDA antagonists are not limited to positive symptoms. Phencyclidine and ketamine (another glutamatergic antagonist), for example, produce negative symptoms and cognitive deficits in verbal declarative memory and executive functions in normal subjects. Furthermore, administration of ketamine to individuals with schizophrenia worsens psychotic symptoms and neuropsychological deficits.

Although there are many reports of dopaminergic and glutamatergic dysfunction in schizophrenia, scientists still debate the nature of these disruptions. One of the major questions regarding the role of these neurotransmitters in schizophrenia is cause or consequence. Because people with schizophrenia are usually unavailable until they become ill, it has been difficult to establish whether the dopaminergic abnormalities reported by scientists come before the illness and contribute to its emergence, or are a consequence of the effects of disease onset, psychosis, or its pharmacological treatments. Studies of non-medicated, first-episode patients have confirmed that these abnormalities are largely in place before illness onset, and get worse with time. Additional longitudinal work currently underway in first-episode patients will need to be evaluated before this conclusion is considered firm.

Research on the biochemical basis of schizophrenia is often done on subjects with either schizophrenia or schizoaffective disorder; thus, results from the two diagnostic categories have not traditionally been reported separately and, unfortunately, the neurochemical basis of schizoaffective disorder has yet to be investigated separately from schizophrenia. As a consequence, our knowledge of what differentiates schizoaffective disorder from schizophrenia at the biochemical level is lacking. The quantity and quality of studies on neurotransmission in schizotypal personality disorder are also less than remarkable.

Schizophrenia research is evolving more and more towards molecular methods, which promise to shed light upon the pathology of the disease and, ultimately, its aetiology. However, the true molecular aetiology of schizophrenia is only slowly being uncovered, and, as is typical, research into the molecular biological bases of schizophrenia-spectrum disorders will likely lag behind. Examination of these disorders at increasingly microscopic levels of analysis, including the genomic levels, will be necessary before their true foundations will be revealed. The challenge for the coming years will be to clarify further the specific pathological proteins that give rise to these disorders as a means to illuminate their common etiologic components. Such data will provide the basis for understanding how environmental and biological factors combine to influence one's placement along the schizophrenia spectrum, and also will facilitate the effective—but targeted—treatment of each condition as a separate entity that dictates a specific management strategy.

9

Is schizophrenia a neurodevelopmental disorder?

> ### → Key points
>
> ◆ Neurodegenerative disorders occur when the causes of a disease attack and degrade a normal brain.
>
> ◆ Neurodevelopmental disorders occur when the causes of a disease stop the brain from developing normally.
>
> ◆ Schizophrenia is a neurodevelopmental disorder, not a neurodegenerative one.
>
> ◆ The relatively late onset of schizophrenia (typically in the late teens and early 20s) may be preceded by years of subtle clues that do not draw clinical attention but are still signs of abnormal neurodevelopment.
>
> ◆ Stress or other environmental factors in early adulthood may bring on the illness in individuals who are put at risk by problems in neurodevelopment.

The research we have discussed suggests that schizophrenia occurs when abnormal genes and environmental risk factors combine to cause brain dysfunction. In the past two decades, several researchers—notably Drs Daniel Weinberger, Larry Seidman, and Patricia Goldman-Rakic—have concluded that schizophrenia is a neurodevelopmental brain disorder. This suggests that schizophrenia emerges because of the way the brain is built early in life.

To understand this concept, consider brain disorders that do not have a neurodevelopmental origin but instead, come about because of the way the brain breaks down after it is developed. We call these disorders neurodegenerative because the causes of the disease attack and degrade a normal brain. The senility of old age, which doctors call dementia, is a common example. When some people age, their brain is degraded by events such as many strokes or the ravages of Alzheimer's disease. After a few years, a person who once functioned normally can no longer do simple tasks. Other examples are acquired brain syndromes, which occur after an injury to the head, and disorders due to the ingestion of toxic substances (e.g., drugs, lead paint). In each of these cases, some external agent has acted on a normal brain to make it abnormal.

In neurodevelopmental disorders, the brain does not develop (i.e., grow) properly. In other words, it was never really normal to begin with. We know that genes contain the 'blueprint' for building the brain. For schizophrenia, this blueprint contains errors so that the brain is not 'built' correctly. Dr Patricia Goldman-Rakic suggested that certain brain cells in individuals with schizophrenia do not 'migrate' correctly during development. That is, normal brain development requires that cells locate themselves in the right spot and connect to one another in specific patterns. In schizophrenia, it may be that some cells are in the wrong place, some do not make necessary connections, and others make connections that should not be made. It is as if the blueprint for a home told the electrician to put the light switch for the kitchen in the living room.

As we discussed before, schizophrenia genes and early environmental risk factors such as pregnancy complications may lead to abnormal brain development. If so, then why does the disorder lie dormant for many years? The average age at onset for schizophrenia is between 18 and 25 years for men and 26–45 years for women. If the brain's blueprint is wrong, shouldn't we see more schizophrenia in childhood?

Schizophrenia researchers are currently seeking detailed answers to these questions. In the meanwhile, we can provide partial answers. First, recall the studies discussed in previous chapters describing children of mothers with schizophrenia as having deviant scores on neuropsychological measures of brain functioning. Drs Barbara Fish and Joseph Marcus showed that among such children, those who eventually developed schizophrenia had measurable neurologic abnormalities. In fact, a recent meta-analysis of similar studies recently concluded that delays in three 'soft' neurological signs (walking, standing unsupported, and sitting unsupported) were early indicators of the later development of the disorder. These studies showed that the brains of individuals with schizophrenia were not normal in childhood, well before the onset of the illness.

The brain abnormalities of children who, much later go on to develop schizophrenia probably impair their functioning at school and make it difficult to form friendships. Dr Elaine Walker collected the home movies made of individuals with schizophrenia when they were children, prior to their first schizophrenic episode. The movies also recorded some children who did not develop schizophrenia. Dr Walker had psychology graduate students and experienced clinicians view these movies with the goal of deciding which children in the movies eventually became affected with schizophrenia. Although they made

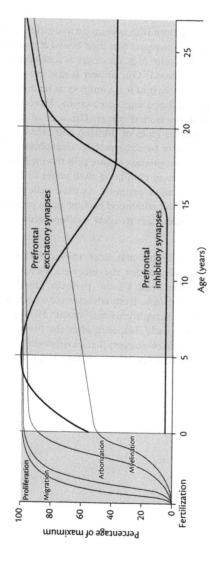

Figure 9.1 Brain Growth in Development.

Reproduced with permission from Insel TR, 'Rethinking schizophrenia', *Nature*, Volume 468, Issue 7321, pp. 187–93, Copyright © 2010 Springer Nature.

some errors, these raters were able to classify many of the children correctly. This study suggests that, although these children would not develop schizophrenia for many years, their social behaviour was unusual enough to be detected by the study's raters.

These studies show that children who later go on to develop schizophrenia show abnormal behaviours, which suggests that their brains at that early point in time were already abnormal. But why does the onset of schizophrenia usually occur in late adolescence or adulthood? One answer is that the brain's development takes some time. Although much of it is complete at birth, the brain continues to develop throughout childhood and adolescence. Moreover, the last part to complete development is the frontal cortex. This area of the brain is involved in some of our most complex types of thinking and behaviour and is one that brain-imaging studies show to be abnormal in schizophrenia. Very early in development, much of the brain produces more cells than will be needed at adulthood. The 'overgrown' brain of childhood then starts to lose unneeded cells as it matures, in a process called 'pruning'. As these cells prune away, and the stresses of late adolescence and adulthood become more pronounced, the faulty architecture of the brain may start to allow schizophrenia symptoms to show (Figure 9.1).

Thus, the onset of schizophrenia may need to wait for certain areas of the brain to develop incorrectly, or for the incorrect development to be 'unmasked'. When these brain areas cannot perform functions necessary for people to cope with the transition from adolescence to adulthood or with the challenges of adulthood, schizophrenia may ensue. However, many patients onset in their late 20s and early 30s, long after the brain has completed its development. These later onsets suggest that environmental factors may need to stress the abnormally developed brain before symptoms of the disorder appear.

10

How is schizophrenia treated?

➲ Key points

◆ Although there is no 'cure' for the disorder, antipsychotic medications can control the positive symptoms of schizophrenia for many patients.

◆ Antipsychotic medications can cause severe side effects, including involuntary movements, restlessness, obesity, and metabolic syndrome.

◆ The largest and most comprehensive studies that compared treatments have found clozapine to be a bit more effective than other antipsychotics, but its use is limited due to a rare but potentially deadly side effect, agranulocytosis.

◆ Psychotherapy is not sufficient to treat schizophrenia on its own but can be useful to help manage social and behavioural problems associated with the disorder.

In earlier chapters, we described the many advances in our understanding of schizophrenia. Unfortunately, we still do not have a detailed blueprint of what exactly goes wrong in the brain in schizophrenia, or a means for 'fixing' the brain. But even without a clear grasp of all the underlying, hidden facts, we have still made many gains. While we search for more clues, we need to use the facts on hand to help individuals with schizophrenia and their families to relieve their suffering. As the saying goes, 'The perfect is the enemy of the good', and some good treatment options exist. So while we work toward a perfect understanding of schizophrenia and develop treatments that are targeted toward each individual's personal form of the disorder, we must rely on the evidence for existing treatments to separate the 'good' from the 'bad'. Bad treatments are those that are ineffective, counterproductive, or have a high risk of very serious side effects. Good treatments are those that have good evidence of helping a fair number of patients to reduce at least the positive symptoms of the disorder while having a relatively low risk of serious side effects. No current treatment for the disorder will work for all affected individuals, and we do not yet have a way of being able to tell before treatment what chance the affected individual has of improving with a given treatment. These are all goals for future research, including the discovery of brand new medicines. For now, we review the currently available treatments with the best evidence of being able to help a good number of patients.

What brings affected individuals to treatment?

The onset of schizophrenia can be frightening, for both affected individuals and their families. Affected individuals begin to express many odd beliefs: that people are trying to harm them—friends, relatives, strangers, or celebrities; that others can hear their thoughts as if spoken aloud; that voices talk to them, even when they are alone. In addition, they cannot express feelings and thoughts clearly and are frustrated by the doubts expressed by relatives and friends. They can sense that something is wrong, but do not see themselves as a patient who needs professional help. Well-meaning relatives and friends may try to reason with them, but such discussions often break down into arguments or heated disputes.

Relatives struggle with the affected individual's bizarre beliefs, unreasonable behaviours, and increasing isolation. When they ask the individual to seek medical help, they are often disappointed. To the individual with schizophrenia, bizarre beliefs reflect reality, not the effects of a brain disease. Some affected individuals seek treatment on their own, but usually for a bizarre reason. For example, one of our patients came to the emergency room asking doctors to remove a radio transmitter from his brain. Another complained to a dentist that the Central Intelligence Agency had put computer chips in her teeth. Another sought relief from the rats that were eating his intestines. In some cases, relatives convince the affected individual that a trip to the family doctor might prove useful.

Even when affected individuals eventually see a doctor, they may become very upset when the doctor suggests a psychiatric consultation. Indeed, relatives, friends, and even the doctor may become seen as persecutors in the individual's delusional systems. At this stage, it is important to try to prevent further deterioration by persuading these individuals to be admitted to hospital for an examination. If they refuse and are dangerous to themselves or others, then involuntary admission through legal commitment procedures may be necessary. The legal commitment process can be slow and frustrating to family members who see the dire need for the affected individual to be hospitalized. Judges understand the urgency of these issues, but their duty to the law requires that they be extremely careful not to take away an individual's right to freedom without clear evidence that the individual is indeed dangerous to themselves or to others.

Treatment begins with diagnosis

When individuals with schizophrenia are extremely upset or when their behaviour is out of control, the doctor may suggest an emergency treatment. By calming the patient, this takes care of the immediate problem and helps the doctor collect the information needed to make a diagnosis. When the diagnosis is complete, the doctor will prepare a treatment plan.

Many individuals with schizophrenia—and even their relatives—become annoyed at the time it takes to make a diagnosis. The doctor will request many medical tests: X-rays, blood tests, and other physical examinations. These are needed to be sure that what look like symptoms of schizophrenia are not due to some other physical illness. It would be a tragic mistake if the doctor did not learn that street drugs, a brain tumour, or some other problem had caused the symptoms because the method of treating these conditions would be different from the treatment of schizophrenia. With the results of laboratory tests, they will rule out any disorders due to causes that can mimic schizophrenia. We use this process of elimination because there is no positive laboratory test for schizophrenia yet.

The diagnostic process takes additional time to examine affected individuals carefully, to find any of the symptoms that are usually associated with typical schizophrenia. At most hospitals, a team of professionals works together to make the diagnosis: social workers enquire about the patient's family life, psychologists give tests of personality and intelligence, doctors and nurses take a detailed medical and family history. Some, or all, of these professionals will talk to friends and family to collect additional information. To many, the team of professionals trying to help the patient is daunting. Their interviews and tests may seem tedious and repetitious. Their roles on the treatment team may be unclear. We suggest that affected individuals and relatives clear up such misunderstandings. Most professionals will be pleased to explain what they do and how it relates to the work of other team members. Having an alliance with one or more members of the treatment team can also ensure that nothing is missed and that the best care is received.

We have found that affected individuals and their relatives often confuse psychologists with psychiatrists. They wonder: Why do I need two doctors? Psychiatrists are medical doctors who have received specialty training in the diagnosis and medical treatment of mental illness. Their training allows them to prescribe drugs and to monitor their effects on their patients' mental and physical systems. Psychologists are not physicians, and, with rare exceptions, cannot prescribe drugs. They are trained to assess psychopathology and its effects on thinking and emotion. They are specially trained to understand core deficits that may impair functioning, and to treat schizophrenia using largely psychological and behavioural techniques.

Throughout the diagnostic process, affected individuals and family members must remember a key point: the treatment of an individual with apparent schizophrenia is unlikely to be successful until a full diagnostic workup is completed. Only then can the treatment team prepare an optimal treatment plan.

Medical treatment

Since schizophrenia is a brain disorder, the reader will not be surprised to learn that its primary medical treatment involves drugs that influence brain functioning. Before we tell you what these drugs are, let us be certain that you know what they are not. Psychiatric drugs are not cures for schizophrenia. Most patients improve; some do not. Few go on to live normal lives: milder symptoms may always remain, and episodes of severe schizophrenia may return. Nevertheless, the quality of life for patients and their families is usually much better with drug treatment than without.

Psychiatric drugs are not 'chemical straitjackets'. We sometimes hear laypeople refer to psychiatric drugs with such pejorative terms. This view portrays medicine as mind control. In the extreme, it accuses psychiatrists of stripping the creativity and individuality away from the individual with schizophrenia, of making them helpless to control their own destinies. But nothing could be further from the truth. Psychiatric medicine adjusts brain functioning to help patients think clearly and better control their lives. Without medical help, the patient's personality disintegrates into a chaotic blend of fear and fantasy. With medical help, recovery can begin.

Neuroleptic drugs

Neuroleptic or **antipsychotic** drugs are a group of medicines that have similar chemical properties. Because of their chemical make-up, they can reduce some symptoms of schizophrenia. Doctors usually prescribe them when the affected individual has active, positive symptoms such as delusions or hallucinations. At this stage, the individual is so out of touch with reality that he or she cannot correctly see that efforts are being made to help them. Neuroleptic drugs help break down the emotional and communication barriers that separate patients from their friends, relatives, and therapists. Since the 1950s, when these drugs were first introduced, worldwide studies have shown their effectiveness in treating schizophrenia symptoms. On average, two-thirds of patients show a significant improvement, and about 25% show no or little improvement.

The doctor's first choice of a neuroleptic drug for a patient will be guided by all the information, both medical and psychological, collected during the diagnostic work-up. In almost all cases, the use of a single type is preferred to a 'cocktail' of several. Of course, additional medicines may be added to deal with other medical problems or even other psychiatric problems such as mood problems or anxiety. Sometimes more than one medication is required to treat schizophrenia. Unfortunately, there is no way for the doctor to be certain that the first choice will be correct. The drug may be ineffective, or the patient may suffer from severe side effects.

In such cases, we urge the affected individual to not give up on medicine but to try another drug. The workings of the brain are complex, and our knowledge about schizophrenia is incomplete. Although the group of neuroleptic medications is similar to one another, where one fails, another may succeed. This is the clinical experience of many psychiatrists. Thus, affected individuals and their families should be neither discouraged nor alarmed if their doctor tries a sequence of medications before relief is achieved and side effects are controlled. This is common in the treatment of schizophrenia since we have no way of knowing which specific neuroleptic will be effective for any given patient.

Neuroleptic side effects

Unfortunately, neuroleptic drugs bring with them the risk of side effects that range in severity from unpleasant to debilitating. In very rare circumstances, death can occur. Usually, these problems are avoided or controlled if the patient remains in the care of a psychiatrist.

We call the most common side effects of neuroleptics '**extrapyramidal**' symptoms because they are due to the action of these drugs on the brain's extrapyramidal system. This neural system helps control movement. The three basic types of extrapyramidal symptoms—**dystonia, akathisia,** and **pseudoparkinsonism**—occur in 40–60% of patients treated with neuroleptics. Dystonic reactions are involuntary muscle contractions, typically involving muscles of the head and face. These muscle contractions are uncomfortable, and sometimes painful. They make the patient feel stiff. Because facial appearance and body posture may be distorted, the patient can be embarrassed in social situations.

Akathisia is a subjective feeling of restlessness. It may be apparent in pacing, rocking from foot to foot, other motor activity, or insomnia. Ranging from mild to extremely irritating, it, like other side effects, may lead patients to stop taking their medicine. Pseudoparkinsonism is a condition that is virtually indistinguishable from the neurological disease called Parkinson's disease. It includes tremors, stiffness, and, sometimes, lack of movement. The patient's face may show little expressiveness as if he were wearing a mask.

The extrapyramidal side effects usually occur within a few days of treatment with neuroleptics. Fortunately, the psychiatrist often can relieve these problems. One approach is to switch to another neuroleptic drug. Another possibility is to treat the individual with drugs that are specifically designed to control the side effects. Affected individuals and their families should discuss these symptoms with the psychiatrist. Two key points must be remembered. First, these side effects are not a worsening of schizophrenia symptoms. They are well-known effects of the neuroleptic drugs themselves. Second, they are usually not a basis for questioning the competence of the psychiatrist. Unfortunately, medical knowledge can predict neither which patients will develop side effects nor how severe these will be.

If neuroleptics are used over a long period, a neurological complication, called **tardive dyskinesia**, may develop. Like extrapyramidal conditions, tardive dyskinesia produces uncontrollable muscle movements, usually of the face. Individuals with tardive dyskinesia repeatedly smack their lips together, stick out their tongue, grimace, and move their chin from side to side. These are not as easily reversed as extrapyramidal symptoms, particularly in older patients. Withdrawal of neuroleptics may stop the dyskinetic movements. However, in some cases, the syndrome will not stop, even when neuroleptic drugs are taken away.

Research suggests that about 20% of neuroleptic-treated patients will develop tardive dyskinesia. However, we have no way of knowing, prior to treatment, which patients will be affected. Thus, neuroleptic treatment must be overseen by a psychiatrist or other physician experienced and skilled in their use. Careful, periodic observations of the patient help the psychiatrist spot tardive dyskinesia in its earliest stages when it is easiest to treat.

Neuroleptic malignant syndrome is a severe side effect of neuroleptic treatment. Fortunately, it is very rare. The clinical signs of the syndrome are fever, a fast heartbeat, muscle stiffness, altered consciousness, abnormal blood pressure, shortness of breath, and sweating. If the psychiatrist suspects neuroleptic malignant syndrome, a blood test will be used to see if it is present. If the affected individual has abnormal levels of specific constituents of blood, then neuroleptic malignant syndrome is likely. Because this syndrome can lead to death, the neuroleptic drug will be taken away from the patient. This will reverse the syndrome.

Low-dose neuroleptic treatment

After realizing that neuroleptic side effects were frequent—and that some were severe—clinical scientists sought to develop new dosing strategies. Their goal was to give patients the smallest amount of neuroleptic that would have a therapeutic effect. The cornerstone of this new treatment philosophy was that, during their lifetime, patients should take only that amount of medicine that was medically necessary.

These scientists quickly learned that excess usage of neuroleptics occurs when the dose needed to help a very ill individual is not reduced after the most severe and distressing symptoms have subsided. When individuals with schizophrenia are very psychotic and agitated, the doctor will usually prescribe a relatively high dose of neuroleptic. However, clinical scientists have shown that these high doses are not always needed after the initial psychosis and agitation goes away. Since these drugs have serious side effects, we cannot justify the extended use of large doses without evidence that lower doses are not effective.

The affected individual and family must understand that before treatment, the doctor cannot know what dose is ideal. Owing to differences in physiology, different people may require very different doses to achieve the same clinical effect. Thus, the doctor who changes doses several times is not being erratic, but merely trying to find the optimal dose.

Ideally, drug treatment should be reduced soon after the initial symptoms are relieved. This long-term treatment, which continues after discharge from the hospital, is often called 'maintenance' treatment because it helps maintain the individual's level of functioning and their place in the community. We emphasize that, although maintenance treatment is very effective, it cannot guarantee that severe symptoms will not return. After 2 years, about half of individuals with schizophrenia who have been on drug maintenance treatment will relapse. This is a sobering statistic, yet it compares favourably with an 84% relapse rate in patients who have not been treated.

During outpatient treatment, two strategies are available: low-dose treatment and intermittent treatment. With a low-dose strategy, patients with schizophrenia are maintained on a dose that is much lower than that initially needed. In some cases, this is as much as 90% less. More intensive treatment is saved for periods of symptom worsening. The maintenance dose of medication that will keep target symptoms at a satisfactory level is highly variable between individuals and, unfortunately, can be found only by trial and error.

The intermittent medication strategy withdraws all medication during periods of remission and uses neuroleptics only when the patient appears to be at risk for relapse. This requires frequent observation of the patient by the family and by clinicians so that early signs of a pending relapse will signal a protective increase in medication. Intermittent medication is not common, as it can lead to deterioration of functioning and relapse in more than 50% of individuals with schizophrenia.

'Atypical' or 'second-generation' antipsychotics

After neuroleptics were in use for a while, the next big breakthrough in the treatment of schizophrenia was the discovery of the so-called atypical or second-generation antipsychotics, such as clozapine, risperidone, olanzapine, quetiapine, sertindole, and ziprasidone. These drugs differ from traditional neuroleptics in several ways. Some of these are advantageous. For example, they have relatively few extrapyramidal side effects and can, therefore, provide relief for patients who cannot tolerate the side effects of other drugs. Patients using these drugs are also less likely to develop tardive dyskinesia. More importantly, these are effective in many individuals who are not helped by other neuroleptics. This is especially true for clozapine, which has the strongest evidence of helping previously treatment-resistant patients. But, like all other antipsychotics before them, these newer drugs do not cure schizophrenia. Nevertheless, it is gratifying to see major improvements in some patients who could not be helped by the first-generation neuroleptics.

Sadly, clozapine use, in particular, can lead to a very serious side effect—agranulocytosis, which increases susceptibility to infections. This is a life-threatening condition that occurs in about 2% of patients after approximately 1 year of clozapine therapy. It is impossible to know who will develop agranulocytosis and who will not, though genetics may play a role. Fortunately, there is a blood test that tells doctors if agranulocytosis is developing. If the affected individual follows through with frequent blood tests, the deaths caused by this side effect can be prevented. However, the blood tests must be regular and frequent. Thus, clozapine cannot be used with individuals who are too ill to comply with these tests.

Another very serious side effect of antipsychotic medication is prolongation of the QTc interval, which refers to a change in the typical electrical activity of the heart. All antipsychotics, with the exception of lurasidone, aripiprazole, paliperidone, and asenapine, have been found to increase the risk for this condition. A less serious, but frequent, side effect of second-generation antipsychotics is weight gain, which is most frequent with olanzapine, and least likely with ziprasidone and lurasidone). Most atypical antipsychotic medications (except amisulpride, paliperidone, sertindole, and iloperidone) increase sedation. Most antipsychotic medications (except aripiprazole, quetiapine, asenapine, chlorpromazine, and iloperidone) also increase prolactin levels, which can lead to sexual dysfunction.

First- and second-generation antipsychotic medications have now been compared and exhaustively evaluated in several clinical trials sponsored by the US government (foremost among these is the Clinical Antipsychotic Trials in Intervention Effectiveness, or CATIE), pharmaceutical companies in the private sector, and elsewhere. A recent meta-analysis of these head-to-head comparisons confirmed that clozapine has a slight advantage in terms of efficacy, but the differences were small and all of these and the first-generation antipsychotics reduce positive symptoms of schizophrenia relative to a placebo treatment. Thus, the data suggest that the psychiatrist and patient can be assured in trying several different treatment options to minimize side effects, without worrying about a major loss of effectiveness in treating symptoms.

Other medical treatments

A number of other medications have been suggested for the treatment of schizophrenia. These are too numerous to be discussed in this book. However, affected individuals and families should know that, although neuroleptics are usually the first choice for treatment, other medicines are available for special cases.

For example, lithium has been shown to be effective in some individuals with schizophrenia. For some patients, lithium may be added to neuroleptic treatment to improve its effectiveness. In some cases, drugs called benzodiazepines (often used to treat anxiety) have been helpful. However, they may worsen symptoms in some individuals with schizophrenia. Drugs known as anticonvulsants (because they prevent convulsions in individuals with epilepsy) sometimes help with schizophrenia. This appears to be especially true for violent individuals with schizophrenia and for those who have abnormal brain waves as measured by the electroencephalogram. However, they do not appear to be effective as a maintenance treatment. In essence, none of these is a useful first-line treatment for schizophrenia but may have some place in helping with mood or anxiety problems that are often seen in the disorder.

Beyond drug treatment, there are additional medical methods that have been tried for reducing the symptoms of schizophrenia. Electroconvulsive therapy is one, known in the popular press as 'electric shock treatment' because it involves the application of an electrical impulse to the affected individual's brain. Electroconvulsive therapy is used for some cases of severe depression; however, it has not proved to be helpful for individuals with schizophrenia. Other types of brain stimulation do show promise for reducing schizophrenia symptoms, however. Foremost among these today are so-called 'deep-brain stimulation' methods, such as repetitive transcranial magnetic stimulation. In this treatment, an individual with schizophrenia undergoes several sessions, usually over the course of a few weeks, in which specific parts of the brain are stimulated by electromagnetic waves. The targeted brain regions typically are those that have been found to be disrupted in schizophrenia, such as frontal cortex. A recent meta-analysis of transcranial magnetic stimulation trials has shown reliable evidence of a reduction in negative symptoms, which are usually resistant to treatment with drugs. This technique also shows a reliable effect on reducing hallucinations, but may actually increase the chance of other positive symptoms.

Overall, transcranial magnetic stimulation does seem to be a useful adjunct to drug treatment for individuals with schizophrenia, especially those with prominent negative symptoms.

Compliance with medical treatment

Obviously, no medication will work well if the affected individual does not take it. Although this is true for all illnesses, it is especially problematic for schizophrenia. The illness makes it difficult—if not impossible—for the affected individual to understand how important these drugs are. Most people will live with the side effects of drugs that reduce the symptoms of an illness. However, the individual with schizophrenia may not be able to correctly weigh the benefits of treatment against the discomfort of side effects. Also, for some individuals with schizophrenia the drug becomes part of their delusion. They may believe that the doctor is trying to poison them or control their mind for evil reasons.

Owing to these problems, nearly half the patients being treated for schizophrenia fail to take their medicine after leaving the hospital. Even when in the hospital, one in five patients does not take the medicine given to them. Failure to take medicine creates a complicated legal, ethical, and medical dilemma. Legally, we cannot force a patient to take medicine or enter a hospital unless the courts determine that the patient is a danger to himself or to others. Ethically, the treatment team ought to provide the best possible treatment. Medically, the best possible treatment is, usually, antipsychotic medication; but patients frequently refuse this alternative.

This dilemma puts clinicians in a helpless situation and frustrates family members. Imagine the anguish of parents who, after seeing their child's psychosis diminish with drug treatment, must watch his condition worsen because he rejects the medicine. There is no simple solution to this dilemma, but we can take steps to avoid it. Our experience shows that doctors, affected individuals, and their families must deal with this problem during the early phases of treatment. In particular, the doctor and the family must work together to help the affected individual continue with the treatment. If one member of the family (or perhaps a friend) has earned the individual's trust more than others, that person should play a major role in planning for treatment compliance. Some individuals with schizophrenia value the advice of a relative or friend much more than that of the doctor.

Of course, friends and family cannot convince the patient to comply with treatment if they do not know why the medicine is so important. Thus, the doctor or other members of the treatment team should spend some time educating them about these issues. The psychiatrist should tell families why they believe the medicine works and what types of side effects may occur. When they understand the costs and benefits of treatment, they can better convey these to their affected family member. Friends and family also need to become good observers of the patient. If we catch the emergence of side effects at an early stage or re-emergence of positive symptoms, we can avoid the compliance problem by switching the individual to a different drug.

Preparing the individual with schizophrenia and their family for compliance does not always work. Such cases call for additional action. First, the doctor should determine if the affected individual is actively refusing medicine or is passively not taking it. This distinction is crucial. For some patients, not taking medicine reflects the negative symptoms of apathy and inactivity. For these individuals, not taking medicine is like not leaving home, not talking with relatives, not dressing, and so on. If this is the case, then the doctor can prescribe a long-acting drug.

Most antipsychotic drugs are given in pills. These are short-acting because their effects wear off quickly when the pills are not taken. In contrast, one dose of a long-acting drug can be effective for many weeks. These long-acting antipsychotic drugs have been prepared so that they are absorbed into the body slowly, exerting a therapeutic effect for a relatively long time. However, they are not available in pill form—they must be injected into the body. Since the patient must go to the doctor's office for the injection, this can be inconvenient. Nevertheless, for some patients, there is no alternative.

Injectable neuroleptics will not always solve a passive non-compliance problem. Since these long-acting drugs are prepared from a very potent type of neuroleptic, they have more side effects than some neuroleptics taken in pill form. In many cases, they are discontinued because the affected individual begins to refuse injections actively or the doctor sees that the side effects are too severe to justify their use.

If the affected individual actively refuses medicine, then the doctor should work with the family to learn the reasons for refusal. Many reasons are possible. Some individuals are annoyed with side effects but never mention this to their doctor or family. Others have delusions that interfere with treatment. For example, one patient believed that the drug was dissolving his internal organs. We have also known patients who think they are cured and that medicine is no longer necessary.

After discovering the reasons for non-compliance, the doctor must establish a plan to try to reverse the patient's decision. In some cases, it is possible to reason with the patient. In others, we can achieve compliance by using a different drug. Unfortunately, many refusals of medication cannot be easily reversed. The patient may simply be too ill to realize that treatment is necessary.

When this occurs, a judge in a court of law must determine if the individual is legally a danger to himself or to others. Although there is no simple definition of danger that applies to all affected individuals, several examples should clarify what is meant. Clearly, the individual who plans to hurt or kill another is a danger to society. Some may have no clear plan, yet will be considered dangerous if their thoughts or behaviour reveal this to be likely.

The suicidal person presents the most obvious case of an affected individual who is dangerous to himself. However, a judge could also reach this conclusion when faced with a non-suicidal individual whose behaviour is likely to lead to injury or death. Some individuals with schizophrenia refuse to eat; others may place themselves in physical danger. For example, a patient who runs in front of traffic at the command of a hallucination is a danger to himself.

We emphasize that the final determination of dangerousness is a legal decision, not a medical one. Although the doctor's opinion will strongly influence a judge's decision, the doctor does not have the authority to treat a non-compliant patient without legal approval. Of course, the authority of the doctor will depend on the legal system where the individual is being treated.

Psychotherapy

Psychological treatment, or psychotherapy, is a very broad term. It refers to any therapeutic approach seeking to change thoughts and behaviour by talking with affected individuals and/or their families. This does not mean that psychological and medical therapies cannot be used at the same time. In fact, for many individuals with schizophrenia, this is the ideal treatment plan. In psychotherapy, the client meets on a regular basis with a therapist to talk about problems that may not be directly related to the causes of schizophrenia. There are many types of psychotherapy, and these differ dramatically. Some have clients recall events from childhood; the therapist says very little but tries to guide clients towards insights about their life and their problems. Other psychotherapies deal only with patients' day-to-day problems; in these, therapists often help patients solve specific problems (e.g., finding a job).

After examining scientific studies of psychotherapy for schizophrenia and other disorders, the American Psychiatric Association Commission on Psychotherapies concluded that, although useful for many other psychiatric problems, psychotherapy was not an effective treatment for schizophrenia on its own. The Commission did not rule out psychotherapy for individuals with schizophrenia, but it clearly indicated that it should be seen as an addition to drug treatment, not a replacement.

In the treatment of schizophrenia, the skills of the psychotherapist are useful in a variety of ways. The development of a productive patient–therapist relationship will foster compliance with drug therapy and motivation for the behavioural and family treatments we discuss later. By helping the patient deal with the social and psychological consequences of schizophrenia, the psychotherapist can become a valuable ally.

Behavioural therapy

Behavioural therapy is different from other psychological treatments in several ways. Unlike many psychotherapies, its goal is to change what patients do (behaviour) using scientific principles of learning discovered by psychologists. Supported by decades of psychology research, these principles describe the laws that govern learning. Behavioural therapists use these laws to change behaviour in their patients.

One prominent class of behavioural therapies is called cognitive behavioural therapy (CBT). CBT is very effective for a range of psychiatric disorders but has only more recently been employed in schizophrenia, where it is presently accepted as a complement to medication management. CBT has been shown to help effectively manage positive and negative symptoms, as well as improve patients' adherence to medication regimens and compliance with medical advice. In some cases, CBT may also improve insight, and reduce aggression. With regard to negative symptoms, CBT in schizophrenia often focuses on the patient's inability to deal with social situations. One goal is to help the patient achieve an ideal level of social activity for them. For example, marked social isolation appears to produce more schizophrenic deterioration. On the other hand, too much social activity may produce an increase in psychotic symptoms. If counsellors and relatives do not understand the need for the affected individual to control social activity and the protective nature of some social withdrawal, they may place too much pressure on the individual to engage in social activities.

The behavioural rehabilitative programme for an individual with schizophrenia must be tailored to the particular problems and concerns of that individual. Many alternatives are available. In what follows, we briefly review three behavioural methods that have been effective in the treatment of schizophrenia: reward and punishment, social skills training, and family therapy.

Reward and punishment

The effects of reward and punishment on behaviour are obvious. We usually do things that are rewarded and avoid activities that are punished. Examples of rewards can be money, products, and social recognition. Punishment can be the withdrawal of a reward or the infliction of physical or emotional harm. Psychology's principles of learning describe how changes in rewards and punishments change behaviour. These principles have been carefully applied to individuals with schizophrenia in a therapeutic programme known as the token economy. The token economy is only useful in treatment settings where affected individuals can be observed for long periods of time. These include hospital wards (where the patient stays overnight), day hospitals (where the individual stays only during the day), and group homes (supervised homes for several affected individuals).

A 'token' is any object that is small and easily identified (e.g., a poker chip). The tokens are used to reward individuals for appropriate behaviour. At first, the tokens are given regardless of behaviour. This is necessary so that the individuals can learn that the tokens have value. This learning occurs because they can use tokens to buy rewards from the staff. These rewards are usually valued items (e.g., special foods) or privileges (e.g., access to the television or game rooms).

The affected individual learns the value of tokens by buying rewards from the staff with the tokens given at the outset of the programme. Eventually, the individual must earn tokens. Tokens are earned according to rules set out by staff in a behavioural programme tailored to each individual. The programme specifies the types and degree of behaviour change required to earn a specified number of tokens.

Token economies can teach appropriate self-care and social behaviours to individuals with schizophrenia. Unfortunately, it is often difficult for the individual to continue these changes after leaving the programme. Another problem with this method is that for clinicians to increase the frequency of desired behaviours, they must see the patient doing the behaviours—even if only rarely. For example, we may wish to teach a very ill patient how to converse with others. If he never talks to others a token economy cannot help. If he talks to others rarely, then by rewarding conversation with tokens, we can increase his level of social conversation. In many cases, the individual will not emit the desired behaviour in any form. This is often the case for social behaviours. Indeed, some affected individuals exhibit very little, if any, appropriate social behaviour. Response acquisition procedures were created to deal with this problem. As the name indicates, these methods help patients acquire a response (i.e., a behaviour) that they do not currently have. Since this work has mostly focused on social behaviours, these techniques are often referred to as social skills training.

Social skills training

Social skills training is usually performed with groups of affected individuals. This creates an artificial social situation that is useful for teaching social behaviour. Although the details of the method vary among hospitals and clinicians, each of these methods shares a common feature: the therapists actively teach the individuals in the group how to use verbal and non-verbal behaviour in social situations.

One programme, developed by Dr James Curran at Brown University, uses groups of three or four affected individuals and two co-therapists. In a typical therapy session, the therapists complete eight tasks. (1) The therapists review the social behaviours that had been learned in the previous session. They also determine whether the group members practised these behaviours outside of the training session. Clearly, social skills training will be useless if individuals do not practise the newly learned behaviour in real social situations. (2) Next, the therapists present a summary of the lesson to be taught during the session. This clarifies what behaviour is to be learned and why it is useful in social situations. (3) Since affected individuals learn best by observation, the therapists perform the skill described in the lesson or present a video of someone doing so. The group members observe the performance and are encouraged to ask questions as needed. (4) Since many individuals with schizophrenia are very passive and will not ask questions, the therapists quiz the group members on what they have observed in order to be certain that they were paying attention to the lesson. (5) Next, it is the group members' turn to practise the newly learned social behaviour. The individuals usually practise in pairs, one pair at a time. Their performance is recorded. (6) The group observes the recorded behaviour of the individuals in the pair. The therapist then leads a discussion designed to provide feedback to the group and to help others learn more about how to practise the skill. (7) After all group members have had an opportunity for feedback, they work in pairs to master the skill with repeated practise. (8) The session ends with the therapists asking the group members to practise the newly learned social skill outside of the therapy session. They usually set a very reasonable goal. For example, they might ask the individuals to practise the skill one time each day.

Behavioural family therapy

Although the family environment does not play a role in the *aetiology* or cause of schizophrenia, it may affect the *course* of the illness. In other words, specific types of family interaction may worsen schizophrenia symptoms and result in increased rates of relapse and hospitalization. Thus, behavioural family therapy assumes that family behaviours have an impact on the course of the illness but does not assume that the illness was directly or indirectly caused by deviant family interaction. Its goal is to reduce stress in the affected individual's life and to encourage the family to participate in the treatment of the illness.

As pioneered by Dr Ian Falloon in Great Britain, there are three major components to behavioural family therapy: education, communication, and problem-solving. The educational component tries to reduce the family's self-blame for the illness. When family members blame themselves for their relative's schizophrenia, tensions, and bad feelings can create an atmosphere that is, psychologically, not healthy for either the affected individual or the family. Once families learn about the biological bases of the illness, they can throw off guilty feelings and be more helpful in the treatment of their affected relative. Understanding biological bases also helps families accept the need for neuroleptic medication. Some people still see psychiatric medicine as a form of restraint that does more harm than good. This incorrect belief can be countered by effective education.

Families are also taught that affected individuals cannot control their schizophrenia symptoms. Telling an individual with schizophrenia to 'stop being paranoid' or complaining that they are 'too lazy' can be harmful. Affected individuals cannot control their paranoid thoughts or the apathy and withdrawal of the negative symptom syndrome. Accusing the affected individual of showing symptoms on purpose adds stress to the patient and frustrates the relative. This clearly leads to a stressful family environment.

Relatives must be taught not to communicate high expectations for social or occupational performance to the affected family member. Many individuals with schizophrenia will never work and never marry. If they do work, it is usually in a relatively low-paying, low-prestige job. Families should be pleased to see a relative with schizophrenia succeed at even the lowest-paying job—that is a real accomplishment for someone with such a disabling illness. Of course, we do not intend to discourage individuals with schizophrenia from achieving their best. Some with milder forms of schizophrenia can achieve much more than the average person with schizophrenia. Our goal here is for both affected individuals and families to set 'reasonable' expectations honestly.

Perhaps most importantly, the families are taught how to identify potential stresses for their affected relative in their home environment. Although we can define stress and give examples from the research literature, its definition is often unique to an individual. Families must learn to be sensitive to the affected individual in this regard. By learning how the affected relative reacts to stress, and by opening up lines of communication, families can lower the stress level and create a healthier environment for recovery.

Of course, opening up lines of communication may not be easy in some families. Many families do not have the communication skills needed to benefit fully from the educational component of treatment. Thus, response acquisition methods are often used to teach these skills. The method of teaching is similar to that described for affected individuals themselves, although it emphasizes those communication skills that are most needed in the family environment. Some families can identify relevant problems but do not have the skills to find and use solutions. Thus, problem-solving family therapies have been used with some success in reducing schizophrenia relapse rates to a clinically significant degree.

Other considerations

Psychological treatments in conjunction with drug treatment may help prevent relapse. In one study a behavioural treatment included social casework designed to assist the affected individuals in coping with their major roles, in job situations, and vocational rehabilitation counselling. Two years after leaving the hospital, 80% of individuals who received neither neuroleptics nor therapy had relapsed. In contrast, only 48% of those receiving medicine only had relapsed.

Individuals who received both therapy and medicine did better than those taking medicine alone; therapy alone reduced the relapse rate of those who had been rehabilitated to the community for 6 months, but after a year it lost its effect except in those patients on active drugs. This study suggested that maximum benefit can be obtained from a combined treatment of medicine and behaviour therapy for at least 1 year after discharge.

It was also found that therapy had improved adjustment and personal relationships in individuals with few schizophrenia symptoms since discharge, but had actually hastened relapse in those patients with severe schizophrenia symptoms. On the basis of this finding, the investigators recommended therapy only for those individuals currently without schizophrenia symptoms. They suggested that behaviour therapy may be harmful to those with severe and overt symptoms because such individuals cannot comprehend the therapy and therefore feel unable to cope with the new challenges it brings.

Indeed, many investigators have confirmed that too vigorous rehabilitation can result in overstimulation and relapse of positive schizophrenia symptoms such as delusions and hallucinations. For example, Dr J.K. Wing and colleagues of the British Medical Research Council Social Psychiatry Research Unit reported in 1964 that delusions and hallucinations re-emerged in a group of chronic individuals with schizophrenia who were put directly into an industrial rehabilitation unit. This could have been prevented by adequate preparation of the affected individuals, for example by encouraging them to participate in the work periods on the ward, followed by sessions in the occupational training unit of the hospital.

Other types of therapy, if not done carefully, may overstimulate the individual and result in the reappearance of positive schizophrenia symptoms. For instance, intense group psychotherapy designed to uncover 'unconscious motivation' and 'role function' may worsen schizophrenia symptoms. Recreational therapy, occupational therapy, group activity, and resocialization therapy are generally useful, but these too may be potential sources of overstimulation, if carried out too vigorously.

On the other hand, other work finds a connection between an understimulating environment, such as the chronic wards of a large mental hospital, and negative schizophrenia symptoms—apathy, lack of initiative, slowness, social isolation, and poverty of speech. Therefore, in treating individuals with schizophrenia one walks a tightrope: understimulation may lead to negative symptoms on one side and overstimulation may lead to positive symptoms on the other. Neuroleptics can provide some protection against overstimulation, but indiscriminate use of the drugs over a long period of time may lead to troublesome neurological complications in some patients. Behavioural therapies may encourage chronically ill individuals to come out from their isolation but can bring on the reappearance of positive symptoms. In treating individuals with schizophrenia one is essentially aiming to provide the optimum conditions for extremely vulnerable people.

Hospitalization

Over the past century, the psychiatric hospital has undergone dramatic changes. Initially, such hospitals were no better than prisons. Patients were physically restrained and, because of lack of medical knowledge, little real treatment was available. Gradually, these warehouses of human turmoil and despair became real hospitals. Patients with schizophrenia received treatment but were rarely helped to a significant degree until neuroleptic medication became available.

For many individuals with schizophrenia, psychiatric hospitalization is, at times, necessary. Hospitalization is used for four basic reasons: diagnostic evaluation, regulation of medication, reduction of danger to the patient or others, and management of acute problems. Rarely is the hospital used for chronic care as in the past. For most patients, lengthy hospitalization has not been found to be more effective than brief hospitalization.

The longer a patient has been in the hospital, the less likely it is that he will want to leave. Lengthy hospital stays can exacerbate negative schizophrenia symptoms and cause an 'institutionalization' syndrome, manifested by loss of interest and initiative, lack of individuality, submissiveness, and deterioration of personal habits. Therefore it is important to reduce the individual's time spent in a psychiatric hospital after the initial phase of positive symptoms is under control. Unless there is a special indication that he should stay, the earlier the discharge, the better. Many studies support the benefits of such early discharge. The family life of the affected individual and his immediate relatives is less disrupted. Today, the trend is towards short hospitalizations with an emphasis on outpatient care.

Of course, this policy of early discharge can be carried too far. It is not advisable to discharge every patient indiscriminately within, say, 2 weeks of admission without proper preparation for his return to the community. The referral of individuals to community care without taking into consideration whether there are available facilities has resulted in increased numbers of individuals with schizophrenia who are homeless or inadequately housed, unemployed, and unable to care for themselves. These unoccupied individuals in the community spend about the same time doing nothing as they did in the chronic wards of mental hospitals. However, unlike the hospitalized patient, the homeless individual in the community is subject to the ravages of crime, poor shelter, and lack of food.

An overemphasis on community care also puts a strain on the members of the affected individual's family. The consequence of these burdens on the relatives has been studied: the relatives of nearly 30% of first-admitted and 60% of previously admitted individuals with schizophrenia had suffered one or more problems which they attributed directly to having to care for their relative. Fortunately, patient and family support groups—such as the National Alliance for the Mentally Ill—can help families cope with the burden of caring for a family member with this and other mental disorders.

While the patient is in hospital receiving treatment for positive symptoms, every effort should be made to evaluate his strengths and weaknesses and those of his key relatives or friends. All available community facilities, such as the mental health clinic, day-care centre, vocational guidance centre, clubhouse, and halfway house, should be assessed. Once the appropriate facility has been chosen, liaison with the staff there and other preparations should be initiated while the patient is still in the hospital. Long-range treatment plans can be built only if such preparations are carefully made. If the patient needs only a short hospital stay, the importance of maintenance drug treatment, particularly after discharge, should be emphasized to both patient and relatives.

Long-term hospital care

Early discharge from hospital may not be possible for some patients. Their positive symptoms may not respond to ordinary doses of neuroleptics, or the side effects may be so severe that constant changes of doses or changes from one type of neuroleptic to another are required. Some patients may need relatively lengthy preparation for discharge because they lack working skills or education. In many cases, patients are poor and may not have the funds needed to resettle in the community. Others may have long-standing negative schizophrenia symptoms with occasional relapses of positive symptoms. Even after those symptoms have been relieved by antipsychotic drugs, the persistence of negative symptoms will prevent them from early reintegration in the community.

Rehabilitation of individuals with chronic schizophrenia

Rehabilitation of individuals with chronic schizophrenia takes time and patience. After the plan and goal have been set up, persistent effort is needed to achieve them. Not only professional skills but also administrative talents are required to carry out the successful rehabilitation of chronic schizophrenia. Rehabilitation involves a gradual progression from working on a simple task in the hospital to more complex tasks in a sheltered workshop outside the hospital, and eventually a return to full employment in the community. We should use all available resources to rehabilitate each affected individual step by step, at their own pace. Compassion, determination, tolerance, and understanding are essential if we are to help these individuals and their families.

Those involved in the care of individuals with schizophrenia should realize that over-enthusiasm, emotional overinvolvement, and disregard for advances in therapeutic methods may be harmful to these individuals and their families. It is necessary to keep in mind that the exact nature of schizophrenia is still unknown. More research is needed to evaluate the effectiveness of the current treatment programs, some of which are blindly accepted and used in routine day-to-day work. Accordingly, careful clinical observations made with a critical mind and an eye open for problems that might need further research are important at this stage. Interdisciplinary cooperation of all professionals—psychiatrists, general practitioners, psychologists, nurses, social workers, occupational therapists, recreational therapists, and counsellors—is vital. Finally, the value of the experience of the affected individuals and their families in coping with schizophrenia should not be underestimated if treatment programmes are to be carried out effectively.

We must again emphasize that although scientists have not yet completed a blueprint describing the causes of schizophrenia, we can still help affected individuals and their families to relieve their suffering.

Schizoaffective disorder

Advances in the treatment of schizophrenia have thus far benefited patients with severe spectrum disorders, such as schizoaffective disorder, far more than they have patients with 'milder' spectrum disorders, such as schizotypal, schizoid, and paranoid personality disorders, or schizotaxia. As expected based on its mood and psychotic features (and its confusability with bipolar disorder and schizophrenia), schizoaffective disorder has been examined most often for responsiveness to both mood-stabilizing and antipsychotic medications. A review of these studies shows a fairly clear treatment regimen for both bipolar and depressive types of schizoaffective disorder. Historically, either typical antipsychotics or lithium alone were used to manage some cases of the bipolar type of schizoaffective disorder, whereas the co-administration of these two drugs was more effective and, thus, preferable. For the treatment of the depressive type of schizoaffective disorder, combined treatment with antipsychotics and antidepressants was not superior to treatment with antipsychotics alone. However, the efficacy of neither of these treatment strategies was ever evaluated in controlled clinical trials. This is of little consequence, however, as these routines are no longer the preferred strategies for the management of the disorder. In fact, a newer generation of medications has supplanted lithium and typical antipsychotic treatments for many affected individuals.

Newer mood stabilizers such as valproate and carbamazepine, and second-generation antipsychotics such as clozapine and risperidone, have for some individuals greater efficacy and, accordingly, their use is increasing, while the use of valium and typical antipsychotics has diminished. For example, divalproex was found to improve global functioning in 75% of individuals with bipolar-type schizoaffective disorder, and very few of these individuals will suffer serious side effects that would cause discontinuation. In those whom it is well tolerated, carbamazepine reduces hospitalization, recurrence, and concomitant psychotropic medication usage, especially among those with depressive-type schizoaffective disorder.

The majority of work on schizoaffective disorder suggests that these newer mood stabilizers and antipsychotics can effectively relieve symptoms alone or in combination for a fair number of patients. Olanzapine is significantly more effective than haloperidol in treating both the depressive and bipolar types of the disorder. In relative terms, olanzapine is most effective in treating those who are currently manic or depressed. Furthermore, the drug is tolerated better than haloperidol, with fewer serious side effects, but the likelihood of weight gain is higher with olanzapine. Ziprasidone also has dose-related efficacy on psychosis symptoms and overall functioning. As a group, the atypical antipsychotics may have better efficacy for schizoaffective disorder than even for schizophrenia itself, possibly owing to their greater affinity for serotonin 1A, 1D, and 2 receptors.

Schizophrenia-spectrum personality disorders

Compared with the literature on treatments for schizophrenia and schizoaffective disorder, there are considerably fewer reports on treatments for schizotypal, schizoid, and paranoid personality disorders. Many studies of pharmacotherapeutic interventions for personality disorders have examined subjects with extensive comorbidity, thus making conclusions regarding the specific personality disorder of interest difficult to interpret (subjects with comorbid schizotypal and borderline personality disorders are perhaps the most frequent among this mixed group of subjects).

Fortunately, while such flawed methods still appear in the scientific literature, overall trends indicate that they are becoming phased out in favour of methodologically sound studies with more 'pure' or 'refined' diagnostic groups. However, such studies are, at present, still rare. As such, we give only a very brief review of the facts gathered to date.

Schizotypal personality disorder

Because schizotypal personality disorder is a complex and (probably) etiologically heterogeneous disorder, it is not likely that one treatment approach will be useful for all patients. More likely, different treatments and combinations of therapies will be the most useful for different presentations of schizotypal personality disorder.

Individuals with schizotypal personality disorder often view their worlds as odd and threatening places; thus, these individuals may require extended courses of treatment. As with most personality disorders, psychotherapeutic intervention is indicated, while the prospect of pharmacotherapy (other than for acute phases of the illness) largely remains an ambitious goal for the future. A meta-analysis from 2012, for example, found that treatment with antipsychotic medication could reduce some of the more psychosis-spectrum symptoms of schizotypal personality disorder, but these medications did not at all improve overall functioning or decrease the severity of the disorder. Rapport and trust between the clinician and affected individual may be difficult to establish in schizotypal personality disorder; yet, these elements are crucial to the success of any therapy. This can be facilitated by establishing a warm, client-centred therapeutic environment in which the affected individual's delusional or inappropriate beliefs are not directly challenged, but instead slowly rationalized.

In light of the frequent occurrence of paranoia and suspiciousness (among other positive symptoms, negative symptoms, and neuropsychological deficits), exploratory psychotherapeutic approaches by themselves are less likely to lead to positive change than are approaches that emphasize supportive and cognitive behavioural therapies. Such approaches often emphasize concrete interim goals and suggest clear ways of attaining them. Because individuals with this disorder are particularly vulnerable to decompensation during times of stress and may experience transient episodes of psychosis, they can also benefit from techniques to facilitate stress reduction (e.g., relaxation techniques, exercise, yoga, and meditation). Fortunately, there is evidence that at least some individuals with schizotypal features are likely to seek treatment in times of stress.

In addition to psychiatric symptoms, other issues should be addressed in therapy, including an understanding of the individual's cognitive strengths and weaknesses. This may help affected individuals confront and cope with long-standing difficulties in their lives. For instance, individuals may present with deficits in attention, verbal memory, or organizational skills that have contributed to failures in a variety of educational, occupational, and social endeavours, and reinforced negative self-images and the experience of performance anxiety. Knowledge of their more limited cognitive capabilities might allow affected individuals to reframe their difficulties in a more benign manner, and also lead to a more realistic selection of personal, educational, and occupational goals.

To some extent, deficits in specific cognitive domains can also be reduced. For example, deficits in the acquisition, organization, and retrieval of information may be reduced by standard procedures for these types of difficulties (e.g., writing information down in a 'memory notebook', use of appointment books, and rehearsal of new information). In addition, social skills training and family therapy may help relieve social anxiety and overcome feelings of isolation from others. Intensive case management and day-hospital admission may also prove helpful—but more costly—treatment approaches.

Although the psychotherapeutic interventions discussed above appear reasonable and appropriate for use in treating schizotypal personality disorder, more research is needed to determine which approaches are most effective. Such studies are still rare at the present time, but one fact that is clear is that little therapeutic change is seen following a course of analytic psychotherapy. Marginally beneficial effects of day hospitals on the outcome of schizotypal personality disorder have also been documented. An intensive treatment regimen consisting of psychodynamically oriented individual and group therapy, art therapy, and daily community meetings for an average of 5.5 months produced little change in global symptoms, but there was a moderate decline in symptoms.

Several studies have looked at the usefulness of medications in treating schizotypal personality disorder, although most investigations employed small numbers of subjects and combined samples of schizotypal and borderline personality disorders. For these reasons, conclusions about the effectiveness of treatment must be conservative. Typical antipsychotics, in particular, have been proposed to reduce positive symptoms or depressed mood in times of acute stress, but the high incidence of adverse side effects may discourage their widespread use at other times, including the more chronic, stable (i.e., non-crisis) phases of the disorder. Other types of medication have shown generally non-specific effects. For example, fluoxetine is commonly tested for efficacy in schizotypal personality disorder, and it has been shown to reduce some symptoms in individuals with schizotypal personality disorder and other comorbid disorders; however, in groups consisting solely of patients with schizotypal personality disorder, these reductions were not significant.

Schizoid personality disorder

As with schizotypal personality disorder, the presentation and presumed causes of schizoid personality disorder are believed to be numerous. The heterogeneity of the disorder, its chronic nature, and its characterization by negative symptoms that do not generally foster an optimal therapeutic atmosphere make this personality disorder particularly difficult to treat. In addition to these limitations, the virtual absence of outcome studies of the disorder means we cannot discern general treatment recommendations; yet, some agreed-upon treatment options are presented below.

The isolation, anhedonia, and restricted affect of schizoid personality disorder can only be reduced under optimal clinical conditions consisting of solid rapport and a stable therapeutic environment in which the patient can learn to rely on the support provided by the clinician, especially during times of crisis. Existing studies have supported the role of CBT in developing social skills and increasing interpersonal sensitivity, while supportive (rather than insightful or interpretive) psychotherapy is generally considered useful. Analytical approaches may not be well tolerated by the patient and should be avoided in favour of practical, goal-oriented therapy. Thus, setting concrete and agreed-upon treatment objectives may help enrich and extend the therapeutic experience. To increase interpersonal skills and overall social motivation, group therapy may be indicated, but only for the most high-functioning patients. Pharmacologic intervention in schizoid personality disorder has not been traditionally advocated, except to attenuate anxiety or depression during crises. However, there is hope that this condition will become a target for to psychopharmacology in the future. The general recommendations provided above have yet to be tested experimentally for efficacy; rather, they are based on practical guidelines that are in desperate need of fortification by the results of clinical outcome studies.

Paranoid personality disorder

Individuals with paranoid personality disorder rarely present themselves for treatment. It should not be surprising, then, that there has been little outcome research to suggest which types of treatment are most effective with this disorder. Research studies that have examined the effects of various treatments on paranoid symptoms have usually done so within the context of other conditions, such as anxiety disorders or post-traumatic stress disorder; thus, studies of 'pure' paranoid personality disorder are almost non-existent. Generally, family or group therapies are ineffective and are not recommended. It is likely that, due to the patient's characteristic mistrust, a supportive, client-centred environment will be the optimal setting for therapeutic change. As with the other schizophrenia-spectrum personality disorders, building rapport is difficult, again due to the fundamentally guarded nature of the disorder. Stability in the therapeutic setting is also critical to increase the patient's trust. As with the delusions of schizotypal personality disorder, it is critical that the clinician remain objective and supportive rather than confrontational when entertaining the patient's paranoid ideas. An honest, practical, goal-oriented approach without presenting too much insightful observation or interpretation may work best with paranoid patients.

Pharmacologic treatment and management of paranoid personality disorder is not widely supported, although certain medications can be useful during the more severe bouts of illness. For example, diazepam can be used to reduce severe anxiety, whereas administration of a neuroleptic or atypical antipsychotic may be indicated if decompensation becomes severe. However, these medications should be used sparingly to prevent the emergence of counter-therapeutic effects as a result of the patient's underlying mistrust and fear of being manipulated.

Summary

Our understanding of the pathology of schizophrenia has advanced greatly over the last century. The last few decades have seen major gains in identifying treatments. This knowledge has had tangible impacts on the disease: inpatient admissions and their length of stay in psychiatric hospitals have steadily decreased, and more affected individuals are managing their illness effectively, especially through the use of psychotropic medication. These advances have also benefitted our understanding of other schizophrenia-spectrum disorders, especially the more severe conditions such as schizoaffective disorder and schizotypal personality disorder.

11

What courses and outcomes are possible in schizophrenia?

⮕ Key points

- Studies of course and outcome support Kraepelin's original conclusions: the course and outcome of schizophrenia are, on the average, worse than those of mood disorders.

- Some individuals with schizophrenia recover from the illness or experience a relatively good outcome.

- The course and outcome of schizophrenia can be modified by environmental factors, such as stress and the family environment.

Kraepelin described one of the core features of schizophrenia to be its progressively worsening course with little chance of recovery. In contrast, mood disorders were thought to have an episodic course with good functioning between bouts of mania and depression, and a relatively good outcome. The ensuing decades of research have painted a more complex picture of the course and outcome of schizophrenia. Most notably, in contrast to Kraepelin's bleak outlook, a fair number of individuals can more or less successfully recover from schizophrenia. Dr Manfred Bleuler, son of Dr Eugen Bleuler, reported a 20-year follow-up of over 200 individuals with schizophrenia excluding those who had either died or shown little psychiatric stability over the previous 5 years. Bleuler noted that one in five patients had recovered to normal levels of social functioning and were free of psychotic symptoms. Furthermore, one in three patients had a relatively good outcome. Thus, while patients still experienced hallucinations and delusions, they showed only mild problems in social functioning and very few visible behavioural problems. These results are quite remarkable given that the study was completed prior to the discovery of antipsychotic medications.

Dr Luc Ciompi was able to follow nearly 300 patients for as long as 50 years after hospitalization. Using Bleuler's categories of outcome, Ciompi found 27% of the patients to be fully recovered, 22% to have mild symptoms, 24% to have moderately severe symptoms, and 18% to have severe symptoms. Nine per cent of the sample had an uncertain outcome. A progressively worsening, gradual, and serious onset was seen in about half of the affected individuals, while a sudden or acute onset of illness with little or no problems in premorbid functioning was found for the rest of the sample. About half of the individuals with schizophrenia had a continuous course of illness, and the remainder had an episodic course. In addition, an episodic course was more likely among patients with acute onset. Acute onset and episodic course were both associated with better long-term outcome.

A study performed by Dr Ming Tsuang and team, known as the Iowa 500 study, followed 186 individuals with schizophrenia, 86 with bipolar disorder, and 212 with major depressive disorder for 35–40 years. As a general index of social competence, the share of each group that went on to marry was found to differ markedly between the groups. For example, while only 21% of individuals with schizophrenia married during the follow-up period, 70% of those with bipolar disorder, 81% of those with major depressive disorder, and 89% of surgical control subjects had done the same. The ability to function outside of a hospital setting was seen in 34% of the individuals with schizophrenia, 69% of those with bipolar disorder, 70% of those with depression, and 90% of the control subjects. In close agreement with these findings, productive occupational functioning was seen in 35% of the individuals with schizophrenia, 67% of those with bipolar disorder, 67% of those with depression, and 88% of the control subjects. Also, the portion of each group with no psychiatric symptoms at follow-up was 20% for individuals with schizophrenia, which is the same proportion noted by Bleuler. However, this figure does not compare favourably with the symptom-free outcomes of 50% for those with bipolar disorder, 61% for those with depression, and 85% for control subjects.

The World Health Organization followed the course of over 1000 psychotic patients for over 2 years. That study found no relationship between diagnosis and the length of the psychotic episode leading the individual to be studied; however, the average length of psychotic episode tended to be longer in schizophrenia. Furthermore, psychosis was more common at follow-up in the sample of individuals with schizophrenia (37%) than in either the bipolar disorder group or the depressed group (26% and 14%, respectively), and individuals with schizophrenia were psychotic for a greater percentage of the 2-year follow-up period than the mood disorder patients were. In sum, the course of illness was more severe for the individuals with schizophrenia.

Overall, studies of course and outcome support Kraepelin's original conclusions: the course and outcome of schizophrenia are, on average, worse than those of mood disorders. However, as these follow-up studies showed, a significant number of patients with schizophrenia recover or experience a relatively good outcome. In fact, favourable outcome may be more common among individuals with schizophrenia than was previously believed. A recent meta-analysis of 50 studies found that an average of 13.5% of affected individuals met the definition of recovery, which was defined as improvements in both symptom and social domains and evidence that improvements in at least one of these two domains had lasted for at least 2 years. A separate meta-analysis found that individuals whose schizophrenia started while they were young had a worse chance of recovery, with more hospitalizations, more negative symptoms, more relapses, poorer social/occupational functioning, and poorer global outcome.

At this time, our understanding of factors that relate to the course of schizophrenia is limited, but some progress has been made. From analyses of the World Health Organization outcome data, it seems that levels of work functioning and social relationships *prior* to the onset of schizophrenia are reliable predictors of outcome after the onset of the disorder. In addition, it has been shown that the presence of mood disorder symptoms during the psychosis of schizophrenia is a favourable sign of a good outcome. This connection was noted by Dr George Vaillant, who saw a connection between symptoms of depression and recovery from schizophrenia in a review of 13 prior studies. He found that 80% of 30 recovered individuals with schizophrenia and 33% of 30 non-recovered individuals with schizophrenia had shown depressive symptoms. Vaillant also found a strong correlation between depressive symptoms and remission of schizophrenia in a 15-year follow-up study. Several studies have found similar results.

Clarifying the contribution of depressive symptoms to the outcome of schizophrenia may be clinically useful because depression is common in the course of schizophrenia. Over a 6- to 12-year span, it has been reported that 57% of individuals with schizophrenia had one or more depressive episode. These depressed patients with schizophrenia had an otherwise typical course of schizophrenia symptoms. Further, their illness did not appear to begin with depressive symptoms and was not episodic. Early studies also found that obsessive or compulsive features (repeated, unwelcome thoughts and behaviours) might be associated with a better course in schizophrenia, but more recent work has suggested just the opposite. This is a crucial distinction to be made since a recent meta-analysis found that 14% of individuals with schizophrenia have such features. Preliminary data suggested that the addition of a serotonin reuptake-blocking medication to typical neuroleptic drugs may be helpful for psychotic patients with obsessive/compulsive features. Further studies are needed to determine whether the presence of such obsessive/compulsive features signal a true subtype of schizophrenia, and to explore the best treatment options.

Whatever knowledge has been gained thus far in describing and predicting the course of schizophrenia is due to the high stability of the schizophrenia diagnosis. The Iowa 500 study showed this fact through a re-evaluation of individuals with schizophrenia over a 35- to 40-year period, in which it was found that 93% of schizophrenia diagnoses were confirmed. Only 4% of patients originally diagnosed with schizophrenia received a diagnosis of a mood disorder at follow-up. Similarly, others have found high diagnostic stability in a prospective follow-up of 19 narrowly defined individuals with schizophrenia, in which no patients were rediagnosed with a mood disorder.

Although the chances of a good outcome or for full remission give reason for hope, most patients will have residual symptoms and deal with a chronic course. Also, premature death in individuals with schizophrenia is higher than in the general population, and much of this increase in mortality is due to suicide. As noted earlier, the second-generation antipsychotic clozapine may lessen the suicide risk in such individuals.

Although psychosocial factors have not been convincingly shown to influence the aetiology of schizophrenia, these factors can influence the course of the disorder. Much of this research has focused on the role of stressful life events. Although some controversy exists over the best definition for a stressful event, most researchers agree that stressful events are those life circumstances that require physical or psychological adaptation on the part of the individual. Life events may be negative, as in the death of a spouse, or positive, as in the birth of a child. According to a recent meta-analysis of 16 studies, stressful life events may increase the risk of schizophrenia onset up to threefold. Patients with schizophrenia who relapse also tend to have more stressful life events than those who do not relapse, although relapse can occur in the absence of such events and remission can be maintained in their presence. More stressful life events are found for relapsing individuals with schizophrenia taking neuroleptic medication than for relapsing individuals with schizophrenia who are drug free. This suggests that the protective effects of neuroleptics and the absence of stressful life events may be additive. That is, the presence of one protective factor may make up for the lack of the other. It is important for affected individuals and clinicians to understand these research studies because they provide clues about how to deal with the illness. For example, some parents of individuals with schizophrenia may think that it is a good idea to put some pressure on their children to motivate them to work harder, make friendships, or reach other goals. But the life stress research shows that this may be counterproductive. More pressure and stress make the illness worse, not better.

Another productive area of research into the psychosocial factors that influence the course and outcome of schizophrenia focuses on the effects of the patient's family environment. Expressed emotion (EE) describes the emotional reactivity of family members in their interactions with an affected individual. We measure EE by observing the degree to which family members criticize, express hostility towards, and are emotionally overinvolved with the affected individual. Drs Vaughn and Leff examined EE as it related to the 9-month relapse rates in 128 individuals with schizophrenia living with their families, and found that 51% of patients in high-EE families relapsed, while only 13% of individuals with schizophrenia in low-EE families did. Furthermore, among individuals with schizophrenia in high-EE families, the risk for relapse was strongly correlated with the amount of time the individual spent in direct contact with the family. In addition, the protective effect of neuroleptic medication differed for affected individuals in low-EE and high-EE families. Among the low-EE group, relapse was unrelated to medication status. In high-EE families, however, the relapse rate for unmedicated individuals with schizophrenia was significantly elevated. This increase in recurrence risk was also associated with increased exposure to other members of the family. Remarkably, 92% of unmedicated individuals with schizophrenia in prolonged contact with high-EE families relapsed, but neuroleptic medication reduced this rate to 53%. Most aspects of Vaughn and Leff's study of a British sample were replicated in a 9-month study of individuals with schizophrenia from California. Notably, the Californian study agreed with the British study in finding that a combination of low family contact and regular medication reduced the negative impact of having a high-EE family. The Californian study, however, found no medication effect for patients having more than 35 hours of contact per week with high-EE families. Subsequent studies designed to reduce EE in families of individuals with schizophrenia have found reduced relapse rates due to this intervention. In fact, a recent meta-analysis of 14 such studies found that a family-based intervention, designed to reduce EE, improved functioning and reduced relapse rates by the end of the intervention, and also led to a reduction in symptoms at a later follow-up.

12

How can affected individuals and their families cope with schizophrenia?

> ## ⊃ Key points
>
> ◆ Individuals with schizophrenia should be in regular contact with their psychiatrist during drug therapy, and should only change that therapy when advised by their psychiatrist.
>
> ◆ Individuals with schizophrenia should work with a social worker and therapist to enhance social, psychological, and occupational functioning.
>
> ◆ Affected individuals and families can help prevent relapse by avoiding stressful situations or parental overinvolvement.

It can be overwhelming to deal with the schizophrenia, either personally or as someone who cares for or about an affected individual. One may also be overwhelmed by trying to digest all the facts that we have shared here about this highly complex disorder. As scientists, we too find it overwhelming to lament how much we still don't know, and how to use what we *do* know to make real change for affected individuals. But having the facts at hand gives some sense of control. It is important, then, to clarify at this stage what affected individuals and their families can do to cope with the disorder, both day to day and in an emergency.

How patients can help themselves

Affected individuals learn to cope with schizophrenia symptoms by trial and error. When they have a worsening of symptoms, they may learn to seek hospital admission rather than resist it. Over time they learn that stopping or changing medication leads to a relapse of positive symptoms. They may be able to adjust the dose of drugs to avoid severe side effects, yet maintain a level that prevents symptom flare-ups.

Clearly, not all individuals with schizophrenia can do this. Nearly half of individuals with schizophrenia who are treated on an outpatient basis fail to take their medication; the relapse rate is high among such patients. Patients should be under continuous supervision by their psychiatrist during drug therapy. Even if they discover how to adjust the drug dose, they should share and discuss these experiences with their psychiatrist and not attempt to make changes on their own.

If the patient finds it difficult to remember to take tablets, long-acting injections of medication are available; one injection works for an average of 2–4 weeks. Patients should faithfully follow their doctor's prescription and receive the injection regularly; with time this can be adjusted as needed.

The family has an important role to play in reminding patients to take medicine regularly or to visit the doctor for injections. This is particularly true if the individual becomes reluctant to follow doctor's orders and relapse seems imminent. In these cases, the family's insistence on taking medication may prevent a full relapse of positive symptoms.

Some individuals with schizophrenia learn to avoid situations that may bring on their delusions or hallucinations. Examples of these include heated discussions of politics or religious experiences, indulging in fantasy daydreams, too-frequent contact with family members, exposure to crowded places, or sights or sounds related to the content of the delusions or hallucinations. If these situations cannot be avoided, affected individuals can increase the dose of medication to prevent the symptoms from recurring. Most patients are alarmed when they first hear hallucinatory voices, but gradually learn to live with them; they may occasionally occur even during medication. Individuals may either learn to ignore the voices or to not be upset by them. In some cases, the individual hears the voices only when alone and unoccupied. These individuals should occupy themselves with routine housework, a hobby, playing a musical instrument, or reading an interesting book, especially if the voices cause distress.

Some individuals with schizophrenia are able to work, and many family members encourage patients to seek gainful employment. Before doing so, the family should consult with the doctor to judge if this is a sound goal for the affected individual. The work that individuals with schizophrenia choose should be well within their skill set. An established 'clubhouse', where affected individuals are treated as contributing 'members', can help in this regard, and give the affected individual a sense of purpose and belonging. They should avoid jobs that are very challenging or stressful. A stable, yet relatively simple job can be very therapeutic for individuals with chronic schizophrenia because it can prevent the development and deterioration of negative symptoms such as apathy, withdrawal, and lack of willpower. Of course, family members must learn what is and what is not stressful for the individual. What seems simple and even relaxing to a family member might be quite challenging and stressful for the individual with schizophrenia.

Furthermore, too much stimulation or intrusion from relatives, friends, or professionals may trigger schizophrenia symptoms. Some affected individuals know when it is time to withdraw from an overstimulating environment in order to prevent recurrence. Families must respect the patient's need to be alone. However, too much social withdrawal may cause negative symptoms to develop or re-emerge. Individuals with schizophrenia who also have good insight can learn from experience to avoid over- or understimulation and tread the narrow path of ideal conditions.

The role of the patient's family

Most individuals with schizophrenia are unable to choose the best conditions to avoid over- or understimulation without some help. By living with schizophrenia, many families gradually learn how best to help their relatives with the disorder. It is usually wise for the affected individual and his relatives to live together again after the initial episode of positive symptoms is over, but this requires a great deal of patience, understanding, compassion, and sacrifice from the relatives.

The individual's first episode of psychotic symptoms often leaves relatives with alternating feelings of shock, hope, and disappointment. The relatives gradually come to realize that schizophrenia is not a short-term problem; it is a lifelong disorder that requires long-term care. When affected individuals are actively psychotic, they cannot make sound judgements. Their relatives may have to take action on their behalf, such as starting legal procedures to commit them to hospital. This may be needed to prevent them from harming themselves or others. Even sometime after the initial phase, individuals with schizophrenia may be unable to understand or agree with their relatives' actions.

Living with an individual with schizophrenia can be very stressful. Relatives may find that their continuous efforts to care for the patient require the sacrifice of their own social lives. This can become too much to bear when the individual shows resentment instead of appreciation. The affected individual's unpredictable behaviour, such as bizarre behaviour, talking to himself, silly laughter, and giggling (particularly in front of other people), embarrasses others. Some relatives cope with this by firmly telling the individual that this sort of behaviour is allowed only in private. They also find there is little point in arguing with the affected individual when he is in the midst of his delusions or hallucinations.

At times individuals with schizophrenia need to isolate themselves to 'recharge their batteries' before resuming social interaction. At such times it is not helpful if relatives try to cajole the patient out of this solitude. Continuous withdrawal and daydreaming, on the other hand, may hasten the development of inertia and apathy. Through experience, those who live with individuals with schizophrenia learn when they should be interrupted and drawn out of their self-imposed isolation.

Some parents feel they are to blame for their child's schizophrenia, and insensitive remarks made by friends or professionals can make matters worse. These feelings of guilt, combined with physical and mental exhaustion in the course of their long-standing emotional burden, can cause real suffering. At this point, parents need to talk and ventilate their feelings to friends and professionals such as social workers, public health nurses, general practitioners, clinical psychologists, and psychiatrists. Sympathetic emotional support may help to reduce tensions, anxiety, guilt, and unhappiness. Unrealistically high expectations on the part of the relatives may lead to disappointment, frustration, and resentment. It is important for relatives to come to terms with the lifelong nature of the battle with schizophrenia and to realize that some affected individuals may never return fully to their previous selves, in spite of continuous medication, psychosocial therapies, and constant rehabilitation efforts. Only when the relatives have accepted a realistic view of the affected individual's condition can realistic goals be set for rehabilitation.

Relatives of individuals with schizophrenia can share their feelings and experiences with others who have similar experiences. By learning from each other and venting their feelings of frustration, they can encourage each other to fight the mental incapacity due to schizophrenia. Through participation in such groups, they may also learn what help is available to them in the community, which professionals are most sympathetic and helpful, and how to help the affected individuals and themselves cope effectively with schizophrenia.

When is professional help needed?

Matters concerning medication should be discussed with the affected individual's psychiatrist, rather than with non-professional people who may point to new, unproven methods of treatment. The psychiatrist will often have the best handle on the scientific backing for proposed treatments. Neither should family members stop drug treatment out of fear that their relative will become addicted. No evidence exists for addiction to these drugs and, as emphasized in this book, the drug treatments for schizophrenia help prevent further relapses.

Professional help is also needed if ever the individual with schizophrenia talks about committing suicide. The affected individual then needs immediate attention because the risk of suicide among those with schizophrenia is high; any sign of attempted suicide requires emergency care. The close relatives of individuals with schizophrenia may also sometimes feel that life is not worth living. Such pessimistic feelings may affect the capacity to cope with daily routines and work or produce physical symptoms such as loss of weight, sleeplessness, loss of appetite, gastrointestinal upset, and dizziness. Thus, relatives with suicidal thoughts should seek immediate professional attention too. It is not easy to be a caregiver for an individual with schizophrenia. At times, caregivers need their own therapy to help them cope with their affected loved one. The maintenance of a social support network is essential

In this chapter, we have discussed some of the ways in which individuals with schizophrenia and their families can help themselves. We could have mentioned only the positive aspects but felt compelled to discuss difficulties that are likely to arise in order to encourage a realistic approach to schizophrenia and its many challenges. The accumulation of knowledge about schizophrenia is making such an approach increasingly possible. With tolerance and understanding, many individuals with schizophrenia and families successfully cope with living with the disorder. As long as affected individuals, with the support of sympathetic and understanding caregivers, can find the narrow path between over- and understimulation, they can successfully avoid recurrence of positive or negative symptoms.

Appendix 1

List of family and patient support groups

Australia

SANE
Mission: Help all Australians affected by mental illness lead a better life.
P.O. Box 226
South Melbourne
Victoria 3205
Tel: 61 3 9682 5933
E-mail: info@sane.org
Web: www.sane.org

Canada

Canadian Mental Health Association
Mission: Promote the mental health of all and supports the resilience and recovery of people experiencing mental illness
500-250 Dundas Street West
Toronto
Ontario M5T 2Z5
E-mail: info@cmha.ca
Web: www.cmha.ca

Schizophrenia Society of Canada
Mission: To improve the quality of life for those affected by schizophrenia and psychosis through education, support programs, public policy and research
100-4 Fort Street
Winnipeg
MB R3C1C4
Tel: 204 786 1616
E-mail: info@schizophrenia.ca
Web: www.schizophrenia.ca

Taiwan

Mental Health Association Taiwan
Mission: To connect civil society and mental health professional organisations with local people to enhance mental health for all.
E-mail: mhat.tw2@gmail.com
Web: http://www.mhat.org.tw/

United Kingdom

MIND
Mission: Provide advice and support to empower anyone experiencing a mental health problem, campaign to improve services, raise awareness, and promote understanding
15–19 Broadway
Stratford
London E15 4BQ
Tel: 020 8519 2122
Infoline: 0300 123 3393
E-mail: supporterservices@mind.org.uk
Web: www.mind.org.uk

Mental Health Foundation
Mission: To help people understand, protect, and sustain their mental health
Colechurch House
1 London Bridge Walk,
London SE1 2SX
Tel: 020 7803 1100
Web: www.mentalhealth.org.uk

Rethink Mental Illness
Mission: Leading the way to a better quality of life for everyone affected by severe mental illness
89 Albert Embankment
London SE1 7TP
Tel: 0845 456 0455
E-mail: info@rethink.org
Web: www.rethink.org

Making Space
Mission: To provide high quality health and social care services that are innovative, responsive, and flexible to each individual's needs and choices
Lyne House
46 Allen Street
Cheshire
Warrington WA2 7JB

Tel: 01925 571 680
E-mail: enquiries@makingspace.co.uk
Web: www.makingspace.co.uk

SANE
Vision: Raise public awareness, excite research, and bring more effective profes-
sional treatment and compassionate care to everyone affected by mental illness
St. Mark's Studies
14 Chillingworth Road
Islington
London N7 8QJ
Tel: 020 3805 1790
SANEline: 0300 304 7000
E-mail: info@sane.org.uk
Web: www.sane.org.uk

United States

National Alliance for the Mentally Ill (NAMI)
Mission: Provide advocacy, education, support, and public awareness so that all
individuals and families affected by mental illness can build better lives.
3803 N. Fairfax Dr., Ste. 100
Arlington
Virginia 22203-3754
Tel: 703 524 7600
Helpline: 800 950 6264
Web: www.nami.org

Mental Health America
Mission: Promoting mental health, preventing mental disorders and achieving
victory over mental illness through advocacy, education, research and services
500 Montgomery Street, Suite 820
Alexandria
Virginia 22314-2971
Tel: 703 684 7722
Web: www.mentalhealthamerica.net

Brain and Behavior Research Foundation
Mission: Alleviating the suffering caused by mental illness by awarding grants
that will lead to advances and breakthroughs in scientific research
90 Park Avenue, 16th Floor
New York
New York 10016
Tel: 646 681 4888
E-mail: info@bbrfoundation.org
Web: www.bbrfoundation.org

Appendix 2

Accessing clinical trials and research studies

CenterWatch

The global source for clinical trials information: offering news, analysis, study grants, career opportunities, and trial listings to professionals and patients

100 N. Washington St., Ste 301
Boston
MA 02114
Tel: 617 948 5100
Toll-Free: (866) 219-3440
E-mail: customerservice@centerwatch.com
Web: www.centerwatch.com

ClinicalTrials.gov

ClinicalTrials.gov is a registry of federally and privately supported clinical trials conducted in the United States and around the world. ClinicalTrials.gov gives you information about a trial's purpose, who may participate, locations, and phone numbers for more details. This information should be used in conjunction with advice from health care professionals.

Contact information:
Web: www.clinicaltrials.gov

BrainDonorProject.org and NIH NeuroBioBank

The NIH-funded NeuroBioBank was established in September 2013 as a national resource for scientists using human post-mortem brain tissue for their research to understand conditions of the nervous system, including schizophrenia. Collection of brains is coordinated through the Brain Donor Project.

Web: neurobiobank.nih.gov/ or braindonorproject.org
Tel: 513 393 7878

Further reading

American Psychiatric Association (2015) *Diagnostic and Statistical Manual of Mental Disorders,* 5th Edition, Text Revision. Washington, DC: American Psychiatric Publishing.

Faraone SV, Tsuang D, Tsuang MT (1999) *Genetics of Mental Disorders: A Guide for Students, Clinicians, and Researchers.* New York, NY: Guilford Press.

Luhrmann TM, Marrow J (2016) *Our Most Troubling Madness: Case Studies in Schizophrenia across Cultures.* Jackson, TN: University of California Press.

Mueser KT, Gingerich S (2006) *The Complete Family Guide to Schizophrenia: Helping Your Loved One Get the Most Out of Life.* New York, NY: Guilford Press.

Mueser KT, Jeste DV (2008) *Clinical Handbook of Schizophrenia.* New York, NY: Guilford Press.

Owen MJ, Sawa A, Mortensen PB (2016) Schizophrenia. *Lancet* 88(10039):86–97.

Saks ER (2007) *The Center Cannot Hold.* New York, NY: Hyperion.

Torrey EF (2013) *Surviving Schizophrenia: A Manual for Families, Patients, and Survivors.* New York, NY: Harper-Collins.

Tsuang MT, Stone WS, Lyons, MJ (2007) *Recognition and Prevention of Major Mental and Substance Use Disorders.* Washington, DC: American Psychiatric Publishing.

Index

Notes vs. indicates a comparison.
Tables and figures are indicated by an italic *t* or *f* following the page number.